LIVING WITH
JUVENILE DIABETES

A Practical Guide for Parents and Caregivers

LIVING WITH JUVENILE DIABETES

A Practical Guide for Parents and Caregivers

VICTORIA PEURRUNG

HATHERLEIGH PRESS
New York

Hatherleigh Press
An Affiliate of W. W. Norton & Company, Inc.
5-22 46th Avenue, Suite 200
Long Island City, NY 11101
1-800-528-2550
www.hatherleighpress.com

DISCLAIMER
This book does not give legal or medical advice.
Always consult your lawyer, doctor, and other professionals.
The names of people who contributed anecdotal material have been changed.

The ideas and suggestions contained in this book are not intended as a
substitute for consulting with a physician. All matters regarding your health
require medical supervision.

Library of Congress Cataloging-in-Publication Data
Peurring, Victoria.
Living with juvenile diabetes : a family guide / Victoria Peurring.
 p. cm.
Includes index.
ISBN 1-57826-057-4 (alk. paper)
 1. Diabetes in children--Popular works. 2. Diabetes--Diet therapy--
 Recipes. I. Title.
RJ420.D5 P48 2000
618.92'462--dc21   00-063374

All Hatherleigh Press titles are available for special promotions and premiums.
For more information, please contact the manager of our Special Sales department.

Designed by Dede Cummings Designs
Printed in Canada on acid-free paper
10 9 8 7 6 5 4 3

AUTHOR'S NOTE

This book is written based entirely on my own experiences, knowledge, discussions with medical professionals and research on diabetes. The medical procedures, exercise programs and nutritional guidelines that I have presented have been successful for my children. No part of this book, however, is intended for anyone's personal medical care without first consulting his or her personal physician.

ACKNOWLEDGEMENTS

I wish to express my deepest thanks to each of the following individuals for their contributions in making this book a reality.

First, I would like to thank my Lord Jesus Christ for giving me the strength to make it through each and every day. A special thanks to my two wonderful children, Jennifer and Joseph, for the patience, love and inspiration they have given me to write this book.

Also, to my husband Joe for all his love, thoughtfulness and support.

I especially want to thank Desmond Schatz, M.D., at the university of Florida, Shands Hospital, for his invaluable medical knowledge and support, as well as for all the time spent in reviewing the entire manuscript.

A very special "thank you" to Pediatric Endocrinologist Dorlinda Varga House, M.D., for her tremendous medical knowledge, editing of the manuscript, suggestions and encouragement.

Thank you to Theo Reed for all the patience, kindness and knowledge she gave me.

A special "thank you" to my friend Nancy Kropp for her encouragement, reviewing of the manuscript, suggestions and wonderful support throughout the writing of the book.

I wish to thank my sister, Donna Sharpe, for all her support and love, and for typing and retyping the manuscript!

Special thanks to my husband's aunt, Frances Safford, for all her love and prayers, and for the kindness she has displayed toward Jennifer and Joseph.

Many thanks to John Davis for all his knowledge and the help he has given me on the computer.

I would like to thank Alan Thicke for his contribution to my book and his continued concern for the cure of diabetes.

Also, to Erin Bromley for her help with the photographs, and to Colonial Photography of Live Oak, Florida.

A heartfelt "thank you" to everyone mentioned: this book would not have been possible without each one of you....

CONTENTS

PREFACE

VICTORIA PEURRUNG HAS WRITTEN a comprehensive manual for parents of children with Type 1 (insulin dependent) diabetes mellitus. *Living with Juvenile Diabetes: A Practical Guide for Parents and Caregivers* is not written from the usual perspective of books about a medical problem, which is how a healthcare professional recommends coping with the problem. This book is written by a parent of two children with Type 1 diabetes. Mrs. Peurrung writes from personal experience about coping with and triumphing over problems caused by diabetes. Her positive attitude and devotion to her children makes for an inspiring story of overcoming adversity. Mrs. Peurrung has chosen to write this book to tell other parents of children with diabetes what she learned about diabetes from books and medical journals, and even more importantly, what she learned about coping with diabetes from her own experiences.

Living with Juvenile Diabetes starts out with a riveting chapter in which the author describes how she felt when her two children each developed diabetes. I was touched by Mrs. Peurrung's emotional description of how she learned to give insulin injections and became comfortable with caring for children with diabetes. This personal perspective drew me into the book and made me want to know how the author ended up dealing with various aspects of diabetes treatment. Through a combination of facts about diabetes and descriptions of the Peurrung family's own method of solving problems, supplemented by photographs, lists, tables and a glossary,

Living with Juvenile Diabetes presents a clear strategy for parents to care for their children with diabetes.

Writing an organized and accurate book about diabetes is not easy. Diabetes affects the afflicted person 24 hours a day. Every piece of food, every type of physical activity and every stressful thought can raise or lower the blood glucose level. *Living with Juvenile Diabetes* covers the types of basic topics that are included in most diabetes manuals, such as insulin injections, blood glucose monitoring, nutrition, and exercise. In addition, the book contains some very practical sections on important topics that are very seldom written about, such as educating teachers and classmates, children's camp, babysitters, supplies, ethnic food recipes, and purchasing and cooking foods. In these chapters, the readers of *Living with Juvenile Diabetes* will benefit from the thoughtful advice of someone who has been there and done that. This book describes how a real parent of real children with diabetes copes with real situations where factors that have a large effect on the blood glucose levels cannot be controlled, so that optimal management of diabetes is difficult. An author must be alert and intelligent to identify and organize the various topics that relate to treatment of diabetes. A reader of this book can either go through the book from beginning to end (which is the way that I recommend that the book be read) or else can use the book as a reference manual and select only particular chapters to read.

Living with Juvenile Diabetes contains a chapter about the important Diabetes Control and Complications Trial, which is the basis for the current emphasis on tight control of diabetes. Every parent of a child with diabetes should become familiar with this study's findings. The book also contains an interesting chapter about future directions in diabetes research. Patients with Type 1 diabetes currently must prick themselves many times each day, either to obtain a drop of blood for the purpose of measuring their blood glucose level, or else to give themselves an insulin injection. The topics discussed in the research chapter soon could become reality for patients and eliminate the need for this often painful and inconvenient puncturing of the skin. Minimally invasive and non-invasive blood glucose monitors and implantable glucose sensors, all of which are being developed currently, will eliminate the need for blood specimens to test blood glucose levels. Currently FDA-approved off–site blood glucose monitors that sample blood from the forearm instead of the fingertip are useful for some patients. Alternate routes of insulin administration, which are being developed currently, could eliminate the need to puncture the skin for repeated injections of insulin. Continuous subcutaneous insulin injection therapy, also known as insulin pump therapy, already has helped to improve the control and simplify the lifestyle of many patients with Type 1 diabetes. Future insulin delivery systems, such as inhaled insulin, oral insulin, nasal insulin, or transdermal insulin, might be well received.

I believe that parents of children with Type 1 diabetes will empathize with Mrs. Peurrung as she tells her captivating story of overcoming adversity. I applaud her for sharing the information and wealth of experience that she has accumulated with readers who are interested in learning how to cope with raising a child with diabetes.

David C. Klonoff, M.D., F.A.C.P.
Director of the Dorothy L. and James E. Frank Diabetes
Research Institute of Mills-Peninsula Health Services
Clinical Professor of Medicine, U.C. San Francisco
Editor-in-Chief, *Diabetes Technology & Therapeutics* Journal

FOREWORD

WHEN VICTORIA PEURRUNG FIRST told me of her
intention to write a book on diabetes, I asked, "Why?" There were
already books about diabetes. Although she had read several of
those herself, none had met her expectations. After all, before the
first of her two children was diagnosed with diabetes in dramatic
fashion, she had never even heard of the disease.

The parents, she said, really need to know so much about the
disease. Most importantly, they need to know how to apply the
knowledge about diabetes so that their children will be able to live
as normal a life as possible. Regulating blood sugar levels in childhood might ensure them fewer complications later in life. In an
area in which instructional texts abound, Victoria's story and practical advice are a tremendous and welcome addition.

Victoria's book has been an evolving work in progress for several years. This story, told from a mother's perspective, concerns diabetes and its impact on one family when both their young
children develop this disease. In some ways, the story is like a jour-
ney. It begins during the first days of Joseph's diagnosis, with ram-
pant feelings of anger and disbelief. Jennifer's onset of diabetes 16
months later seemed improbable and even more devastating. Every
day's devotion, dedication and hard work have helped the family
successfully deal with this disease. Energies have been channeled
appropriately in this book.

The Peurrung family had received instruction initially at diagnosis and continues to receive instruction. In taking care of her

children, though, most of Victoria's training has been on-the-job, learning to cope with her children's daily lives.

Parenthood is, in itself, a challenge. Adding the tasks of coping with diabetes makes that job even harder. Victoria has harnessed her experiences and provided an easy and practical approach to caregivers and parents of children with diabetes.

This book is comprehensive, informative and practical. In addition to the more routine management topics, there are excellent chapters relating to the care of your children in school, how to find good babysitters, exercise ideas and nutrition information. The encouraging results of the DCCT (Diabetes Control and Complications Trial), relating good control to the prevention of complications, are discussed, and there are chapters related to exciting research that is being undertaken and which is aimed at the prediction and ultimate prevention of diabetes.

This book is filled with valuable and practical information and is written in an easy-to-understand manner. It offers suggestions to help caregivers modify their routines and organize their approach in daily diabetes care. Many approaches to the care of children with diabetes have been quite successful. Diabetes needs not diminish the quality of a child's life. When caring and supportive parents "reframe" their outlook, their children can begin to hear that it is possible to live a healthy, productive and successful life.

Desmond Schatz, M.D.
Professor of Pediatric Endocrinology
University of Florida, Shands Hospital

LIVING WITH
JUVENILE DIABETES

A Practical Guide for Parents and Caregivers

1

My story
The devastating news

ARLY ONE MORNING AFTER MY HUSBAND had gone to work, I heard my baby Joseph crying for me. A mother knows her baby's cry, and this cry was one I had never heard before. I ran to his room. Fear gripped me when I saw him. His whole mouth, lips, feet and fingers were completely blue. It looked as though someone had smashed them in a door. I was so frightened I was speechless. My mind begged for an answer. What was happening to my baby? I reached for him and the terror spread through me like a wave. Why was his little body cold and clammy? I was overcome by fear. Was he dying?

In an instant my mind flashed back to my wedding day. It was a hot summer day in Florida when Joe and I were married. We were young and in love. Our dream was to marry and have two healthy children. That dream did not become a reality for eleven long years.

On June 22, 1988, God blessed us with our daughter, Jennifer. She was perfect in every way. Two years later, another baby was on the way. Our family would be complete, just the way I always imagined. Our son Joseph was born on December 6, 1990. He was a happy and healthy baby until the nightmare began.

In February of 1992, both of the children were ill. They started vomiting profusely. Within eight hours they became so dehydrated that they had to be admitted into the hospital. The diagnosis was rotavirus, a common contagious gastrointestinal virus. Joseph had an IV in his foot for 24 hours to receive intravenous fluids. Still, he was able to return home the next day. Not Jennifer; she was getting worse. She had to be rushed to Shands Hospital at the University of Florida in Gainesville. Finally, after one week, Jennifer was well enough to return home.

Our children stayed healthy for seven months. On August 30, 1992, when Joseph was only 21 months old, his appetite started diminishing rapidly. I felt that was quite odd, because Joseph loved to eat. So, by the end of the day when he had not eaten much of anything, I called his doctor.

The doctor asked, "Is he drinking and urinating?"

"Yes," I replied.

The doctor said, "He probably has a stomach virus that's going around. As long as he's drinking, he'll be fine."

"Okay," I said.

Two days went by without Joseph eating. I called the doctor again. The doctor reiterated his message: if Joseph had no fever or vomiting and was drinking well and urinating, we were not to worry.

Four days now had elapsed and still there were no signs of improvement in Joseph. Something was wrong with my baby, but what? That night, Joseph was extremely thirsty. He urinated constantly. He would not just wet his diaper now, but also his clothes and the bedding.

His bed had puddles of urine in it. I used a box of diapers and six sheets throughout the night. In the early morning, Joseph was tired and began crying again. I ran to his room and, as I looked down at him, his whole mouth, lips, fingers and feet were completely blue again. His body was cold and clammy as I held him close to me. I was so frightened and overcome with fear. Joe had already gone to work. Who would I get to help me now?

I called my friend Lois to help me. Joseph was shaking severely. We quickly wrapped him in a blanket and a jacket. His little fingers, toes and lips were still blue. Joseph asked for some juice. He had an extreme thirst, consuming 38 ounces within a few minutes.

Ten minutes passed and the blue color began to fade. Lois and I felt relieved to see him looking like his normal self again.

Still, I knew something was very wrong. I called the doctor, who told me to bring him in. He said it sounded like a lack of oxygen. We hurried to the doctor's office.

The doctor came in and examined him. He said, "He looks fine. He just has the flu."

I looked at the doctor as though he were crazy. "I'm sorry, but this is not the flu," I insisted. "He drinks like he has never drunk before in his life. He urinates a flood and you say nothing is wrong with him? Come on!"

His expression changed quickly. "Oh, God," he said, "it sounds like sugar. Just wait here."

Two minutes became an eternity as I waited. I held Joseph in my arms.

The doctor returned to prick Joseph's finger. "I need to check his blood," he said. He pricked my son's finger, then handed the blood strip to a nurse to insert into a meter.

Next I heard the doctor yelling at the nurse. "Don't you know how to operate this machine!"

What was wrong?

The doctor, still in a loud voice, said, "I'll test my own blood sugar level." His blood sugar read 73 mg/dl; the meter could only go as high as 400 mg/dl. Apparently Joseph's had gone to the top. The doctor rushed back into the examining room.

"There might be something wrong with your son's sugar level. We must take some vials of blood from him so we can send them to the hospital immediately," he said. The doctor seemed urgent now, ordering us to go home. "Gather his clothes," he said. "If I'm right, Joseph will need to be admitted to the hospital at once. Just go home and wait for my call."

I felt numb and confused. Why was the doctor talking so fast? My eyes filled with tears; my heart shattered. Why my baby? "No. No. Please, God, let him be wrong," I prayed.

I rushed to the phone. I needed to talk to my husband. When I heard his voice, I broke down and began crying so hard that he could not understand me.

I drove home frightened and alone. What was going to happen to my baby? I could not control my pain; the tears would not stop.

It took me a long 20-minute drive before I got home. There was something peaceful about coming into our yard. I breathed a sigh of relief. They were wrong. When the doctor calls he will tell us they have made a mistake. Joseph is fine. Again I drew deep breaths. Joseph is fine, I thought.

I sat in the rocker cradling Joseph until my husband came home. He wrapped his arms around us, as only a husband could do. We were in this embrace when the phone rang.

Now my confidence left me. I was terrified to answer the phone. It rang several times. Then I picked the receiver up.

"Hello, Mrs. Peurrung, I have some bad news," the doctor said gravely. My ears were ringing. I thought I would faint. "Joseph's sugar reading is over 800, and he is in great danger. He is very ill. You must get him to the hospital now. I am sending an ambulance to your home."

"Wait. Wait!" I screamed. "What does all this mean? His sugar is high? What does that mean?"

"Mrs. Peurrung, your son must get to the hospital at once; your son has juvenile diabetes. We'll answer your questions there. An ambulance is on the way."

"An ambulance!" I cried.

My husband took the phone from me. He told the doctor we would drive Joseph ourselves. We lived way out in the country and by the time an ambulance would arrive, we could be halfway there.

The hospital was fifty miles away. We left immediately. It was a long hour. My husband drove fast, yet carefully. We both felt that Joseph looked fine. We agreed that he did not have juvenile diabetes. No one in our families had diabetes. Most likely the flu had caused his sugar level to rise. We both began to relax with our false hope.

When we arrived at the hospital emergency room, there was a room waiting for Joseph. When the nurses put him in a crib, I cringed. It looked like a cage. We sat there for about five minutes before half a dozen doctors came in.

One doctor was a pediatric endocrinologist; the others were in various stages of training. They wanted to draw blood. It was difficult because they couldn't find his veins. Joseph screamed and cried. My poor baby finally fell into an exhausted sleep.

Joe and I were sitting in the back of the room when the doctor decided to acknowledge us and explain the problem. "Joseph has juvenile diabetes. He is a very sick little boy. His glucose count is 869 mg/dl and he has an extremely large amount of ketones."

"What is juvenile diabetes?" I asked. "I don't even know anyone who has juvenile diabetes. No one in our family has this. Why does he have it?"

The doctor explained to us that one out of 300 children is diagnosed with juvenile diabetes. The medical profession still does not know exactly what triggers this disease. He told us that we must accept it and start learning how to take care of him. The doctor was generous with his time and spent about an hour explaining things to us.

When they left us alone Joe said, "I don't believe them. They could be wrong." This gave us a little hope.

Maybe Joe was right and the doctors were wrong. Maybe after a week or so our baby would be fine. My prayer was that the doctor had given us the wrong diagnosis; but, in my heart, I knew it wasn't just the flu.

I spent the night with my baby. I held his hands all night. Why Joseph? I kept asking myself. He is such an innocent child to be so sick. How will I be able to care for him? I don't know what to do, how to give an injection. I know absolutely nothing about diabetes. The night went by extremely slowly. The morning finally came and I thought things might have changed, but they had not. Joseph had juvenile diabetes, period.

A diabetes nurse educator came in later that morning when the doctors arrived. She tried to explain all about diabetes. It was overwhelming.

"How will I be able to understand all this in just a few days?" I asked.

Clinically cool, she said, "Oh, you will."

Easy for you to say, I thought. Numbly, I reached out as she handed me some papers and a book. There was no way I could do all this. I was afraid and angry. What if I could not care for Joseph properly? I knew that my husband, Joe, couldn't handle this disease. Joe didn't even want to look at a single paper about diabetes. He didn't want to help at all, because he was afraid. He couldn't come to terms with the fact that his young son had diabetes. Without Joe, I was totally alone, isolated and afraid.

At long last, my sister Donna walked into the hospital room. She grabbed me and held me. I dissolved into tears, realizing I wasn't alone. It felt so good to see her. No one else in my family had come. Why are families so detached when you need them the most?

Donna was filled with encouragement. She was very uplifting, but my grief was beyond words. Donna stayed cheerful and tried to make me laugh.

Then the nurse came in. She told me I would have to give Joseph a shot in his leg. "I can't do it," I said.

"Yes, you can," she replied.

My heart dropped and I began to shake. The nurse filled the syringe. She handed it to me.

"Pinch up the skin, insert the needle, push down, then pull out," she replied.

Oh! How can I do this? Didn't nurses go to school first? Do they just expect me to start stabbing my baby with this sharp needle?

I inhaled and prayed, Lord, please help me. It took two nurses and my sister to hold him down. I pinched his thigh and inserted the syringe. The needle dangled there until I yelled, "I can't. I just can't do this." The needle fell from his leg.

The nurse was calm but firm. "You must try again," she said.

Joseph was screaming and screaming. I was crying and crying. "I can't do it!"

"Yes, you can."

I tried again. This time I only pushed the syringe in halfway, pulled it out and threw it on the floor. "Forget it; I just cannot do this."

I ran out of the room crying. In the hallway I tried to compose myself, but it took about twenty minutes before I could return to the room. The nurse took pity on me. She said I could try again tomorrow. Little did she know that I had decided not to even try again. I could not do this alone; I would not do this. Joe was going to have to help me!

I could not stop crying. Every time I looked at Joseph the tears poured from my broken heart. Why my baby?

The room was closing in on me. I asked my sister to watch him. I had to go for a walk. I had to get out of that room.

Walking calmed me. I noticed a young woman standing alone in the hallway. She was crying. I wiped my own tears away. "Are you all right?" I asked.

She looked at me with hopelessness in her eyes. She said, "I don't know what is going to happen to my life next."

"What do you mean?" I asked.

"Well, see my little baby in there? She is only eighteen months old, and this is her second open-heart surgery. But now they have diagnosed her with terminal cancer. She won't see her second birthday. Her father left us because he couldn't take the pressure."

I embraced her. Her plight was so sad. My heart ached for her. She turned and left when the doctor called her name.

My attitude started to change then. I felt fortunate that Joseph only had diabetes.

I continued my walk and came upon a room with children playing. There were at least ten children in the room.

A nurse was in there, as well as some parents. Looking around, I noticed that some children had no hair, some had little hair, and some had baseball caps on their heads. I asked the nurse what was wrong with these children, and she said, "They all have cancer." It was heartbreaking. The emotions I felt for these children were so overwhelming. I ran out of the room and down the hall where there was a room I entered. I was all alone in this small dark room. I started beating the wall yelling. "Why? Why? Why are all these little children so sick and dying?" My back hit the wall and I slid down and sat on the floor weeping and weeping. As I was sitting there, I felt somehow relieved. I started feeling how lucky I was that my baby was going to live a happy life and that I would be able to be part of his life. I knew that God gave me the two children I asked for, and that he would give me the strength I needed to raise these children. I felt so much better. Seeing those other sick children made me realize how fortunate I was. I was coming to terms with the situation: Joseph did have diabetes. I knew if I did not take care of him, he would die. I had no choice but to face it and do the best I could do.

When I got back to the room, my sister and the nurse were there. I told the nurse that I was ready to learn all I needed to know about giving an injection. So she suggested that I practice on Donna. It took Donna and me about an hour to get up enough nerve to prick our own fingers. Once we got past the finger-pricking stage, it was time to advance to giving an injection. We laughed at each other, because we had never realized how chicken we really were. When Donna finally let me give her an injection, she told me to hurry up and get it over with, but what she did not know was that I had already given it to her. This helped me to overcome the fear that I had of hurting my son.

After seven days in the hospital, Joseph finally got to leave. We were glad to be home!

Still, I felt as though I didn't know much of anything about diabetes. I was scared and lost. We had to call the doctor all the time about everything for four weeks. My husband would not prick Joseph's finger or give him an injection. I would get so upset at him because I had to sit in a chair and put Joseph's legs between mine, holding his chest so he wouldn't move, and give him his injection. Joseph would scream and scream. He made me feel so awful. It would just make me cry. I hated to do it, but I had no choice. No one else would help me—and I mean no one.

Joe and I would argue because he would not do anything that had to do with diabetes. He would not read about it, go to the clinic with me, prick Joseph's finger, or give him an injection. Joe was just too afraid. But I felt that if I could do it, he could also. The excuse Joe would use is that he was too tired because "he had worked all day." I felt trapped, alone, and very depressed. The future certainly did not look like a very happy one.

When I went grocery shopping it took me $3\frac{1}{2}$ hours. I had to read labels to know the ingredients in everything. It was a chore just to find the right foods that we could eat. Almost everything had too much sugar in it. But after a while, I began to feel that our family would be much healthier by eating more nutritious foods.

~ ~ ~

OUR DAUGHTER JENNIFER, who was terrified of needles, felt bad that her brother had to have his finger pricked five or more times a day and had to receive two injections a day. When I would take Jennifer to the doctor's office for a shot, she would cry for twenty minutes. I always said how blessed I was that Jennifer didn't have diabetes.

Ever since my daughter was born, she had always been easy to please and quite patient. She was not a demanding child at all. If she wanted something and I was busy at the time, she would just wait until I could get it for her.

Then in January of 1994, $5\frac{1}{2}$-year-old Jennifer came down with the chicken pox. It lasted for about a week, and then Jennifer started to feel poorly again. That night she did not want to eat dinner and wanted to go to bed at six p.m. I thought, Great, now she has the flu. Around ten that night, Jennifer called for me and asked me for some milk. That was quite odd, I thought, because she doesn't like milk. So I gave her an 8-ounce glassful, and she said she wanted more. I gave her more.

"Are you feeling all right?" I asked her.

She replied, "I feel okay." She did not have a fever and looked all right. I went back to bed. At around 11:30, Jennifer called me again. She wanted more milk, so I gave her another glass. At one, again she asked for something to drink. By this time I was getting a little upset. I told her, "It's time to go to sleep, and if you keep drinking like this you will wet the bed."

"I'm just thirsty, mommy," she replied.

This went on every hour until four. Then, as I lay in the bed, I felt that I should check her blood sugar level. I fought with myself for about 30 minutes saying, "No! No! It just can't be. She couldn't have diabetes." I was terrified of the thought of her having diabetes. I didn't want to get up and check her sugar level, but I finally did get up, got the meter, and walked into her room. I didn't even wake her, but I grabbed one of her fingers and pricked it.

She woke up crying. She asked, "Mommy, what are you doing?"

"It's okay, honey, go back to sleep," I said. The count of forty-five seconds seemed like five hours. Then the meter beeped and her blood glucose level indicated 559 mg/dl. My hands turned numb; my heart started beating so fast that I thought that I wouldn't even make it across the room. I ran into our bedroom and yelled, "Oh, my God, Joe!"

Joe woke up from a sound sleep. He said, "What happened? What happened?" I couldn't even talk.

He held me and I said, "It's Jennifer—she has it, too."

"Has what, honey?" he asked, very frightened.

"Diabetes! She has diabetes. It's happening all over again."

Joe said, "No, it's got to be wrong." We both just held each other and cried. We were in such a state of shock. We had feelings of such hopelessness. Why both of our little children? Why?

On the way to the hospital, I held Jennifer and was afraid of how this would affect her now and later in her young life. Even though we were all together in the car, I felt alone again. I knew that our lives would become even more difficult. It was extremely stressful to have one child with diabetes, and now both of my children have it.

The diagnosis was what we thought – Jennifer did have diabetes. The doctor told us that our second child had a 5–percent chance of developing diabetes. But this was not told to us until Jennifer was diagnosed with the disease.... Well, maybe it was, and I blocked it.

Jennifer reacted remarkably well to her diagnosis. The injections were difficult for about two months, and then they got a little easier. By 2½ months, Jennifer started checking her own blood sugars. We were so very proud of her! We never forced her—she did it all on her own.

The night Jennifer was diagnosed with diabetes was the time when Joe truly came to terms within himself about the disease. He finally started helping me give injections and checking the children's sugar levels. Joe's support and love have helped our family come through these hard times.

~ ~ ~

ONCE THE SHOCK of the diagnosis had worn off, the reality of the everyday task began. In our case it happened twice; we got a double dose of reality. I am not going to tell you that it was or is easy, because it is not. It takes a lot of time, patience, understanding and love to raise two small children with diabetes. There have been times when I just wanted to quit.

What made me want to quit was that I knew I was doing everything within my power to keep them healthy and still their sugar levels were either too high or too low.

With time and the doctors' help, the children's blood sugar levels became a little more consistent.

It was extremely hard for me to determine why the children were acting up. Was it because their blood sugars were too high or too low? Or was this just another challenging but normal toddler behavior?

Keeping a balance was my greatest challenge. With juvenile diabetes the usual rules do not apply, as Joe and I learned one morning.

Both of the children were at the breakfast table eating their morning snacks. I was with them in the kitchen so I could see them. They were happy, both eating and laughing. This made me happy, too.

Then Jennifer spilled her drink everywhere. She stopped laughing and sat on the floor.

I went to her, asking, "What's the matter?"

"I don't know." Her tone was hateful.

Joe overheard her nasty remark. He told Jennifer to go to her room. She stood and went into the living room instead.

Joe was baffled. Why was she acting like this? It was not like Jennifer to be disobedient. He went to her and, in a stern voice, he insisted that she go to her room.

Jennifer ran to her room.

Joe followed her. She was sitting on her bed crying. He tried to talk with her to encourage her to tell him what was wrong. She would not listen. Then Joe lost his cool. "Jennifer, stop crying!" he yelled.

In an instant he yelled for me. "Vicki, hurry. Hurry up! Something is wrong with Jennifer. She is looking right through me." I grabbed the glucose meter and some juice and rushed to them. I took her sugar level; it was very low. I had to coax her to drink some juice and eat some crackers. It took about 35 minutes for her to recover completely.

When the crisis passed we talked with Jennifer about what had happened. She was shocked. She could not believe what had happened, nor did she remember spilling her drink, yelling at us or any of the events. To this day, Jennifer insists those things never happened.

This crisis taught us a lot. At the time of the incident Jennifer was incoherent. She was very close to being unconscious or having a seizure. Joe felt bad about scolding her and not being able to see what was happening to her. We both felt guilty. It took us days to get over this incident and to learn from it.

From that day on, we always ask ourselves: Are the children acting up because they have a blood sugar problem or because they are just kids? If we are not sure what is going on with them, we check their blood sugar first and deal with them accordingly.

It is one thing to deal with normal childhood behavior, but

blood sugar swings are stressful for all of us. This situation is difficult to handle. One minute the children can be laughing, having a
great time, and the next minute, a sugar fluctuation occurs and
things can be almost out of control.

As the Boy Scout motto recommends, I've learned always to
be prepared.

I remember one afternoon in particular when I took the children horseback riding. It was just after lunch, and Jennifer's blood
sugar tested at 325 mg/dl. I gave her an injection, with one unit of
regular insulin. The fact that she had eaten only half of her lunch
concerned me. I could not get her to eat more, but she had plenty
to drink so I felt she would be fine until snack time.

We rode the horse around the house. We had been outside for
about an hour. Jennifer said that her legs were shaking as she was
sitting on the grass. I did not think her blood sugar level was low
because at lunch it was so high.

Since we were just a short distance from the house, I was not
too concerned that I had not brought any glucose or sugar foods
with us. I would soon learn another valuable lesson about managing juvenile diabetes.

Jennifer started to cry. Quickly I put her on the horse with her
brother, then guided them straight to the house. Jennifer jumped
from the horse and fell to the ground. I ran inside the house for
some juice and the meter.

By the time I returned to her, she could hardly drink her juice.
She kept crying, "I can't, I can't." Immediately I checked her blood
sugar level; it was very low; 32 mg/dl. As she drank, she slowly returned to normal.

Now I never leave the house without some glucose tablets or
a juice drink. It is just too dangerous to go anywhere without an
emergency kit of food.

Coping with juvenile diabetes is an ongoing education. Just an
ordinary experience such as taking the children and their friends
to the country club pool for an afternoon of splashing and fun can
change dramatically in a moment.

In the back of my mind I was always afraid of their having a seizure, and I kept the glucagon kit close whenever we were away from the house, always hoping that I would never have to use it.

But one sunny day at the pool turned frightening immediately after our picnic lunch.

I put sun block lotion on the children. When it was Jennifer's turn for me to apply the lotion, she shrugged me away.

At first I thought she was just being contrary. Still, I took a mental inventory. She had eaten a snack at 11 a.m. and her blood sugar level tested 144 prior to leaving the house. She was just now eating lunch and had not been in the pool yet, so everything should be okay. Yet each time I tried to touch her with the lotion, she fidgeted away.

She did the opposite of everything I told her to do. I told her that we needed to check her sugar level. I asked her to come down by the porch where there were fewer children. Instead of doing what I asked of her, she went into the pool. I ordered her from the pool. She staggered toward me. It was like watching a movie of a drunk person trying to act sober. She crashed into the chairs, she tripped over her own feet, and there was a blank stare in her eyes.

I yelled for her to sit down. At that point my worst fears surfaced. I dropped the emergency kit and grabbed her. She tried to push me away. We were both on the ground. I struggled with the emergency kit, trying to get some glucose tablets. I couldn't unzip the kit and hold her down, too. I was shaking with fright. How could I do this by myself? No one at the pool offered to help.

Finally I opened the kit and the tablets spilled all over the place. I grabbed one and tried to get Jennifer to eat the tablet. She tried, but it dribbled down her chin. She could not swallow. This is common during a seizure. I tried other things; still she could not swallow. I knew that I had to use the thing I feared the most, and that was the glucagon emergency kit.

It is frightening to learn on the scene, with your child in trouble. It was difficult to work with one hand as I had to hold Jennifer down with the other hand. To administer the glucagon I would need to unseal the bottle, inject the syringe fluid into the glucagon, remove the syringe, shake the bottle, then reinsert the syringe for a dose of medicine. In my panic all I could withdraw was air. I simply could not get any fluid. I started to cry. My child was kicking and screaming. The other people at the pool were staring at us. Still, no one tried to help. I thought, There is no way I can do this alone.

Then I looked at my daughter and knew I had to make the glucagon work. At that point I wrapped my legs around her to lock her down and free both my hands. I stuck the syringe back into the glucagon solution and was able to get only a quarter of solution and a lot of air. With the needle pointed up I removed the air, reinserted the needle and withdrew a proper amount of medicine.

Next I injected Jennifer with the medicine. She screamed and pulled away. All I could do then was hold her and comfort her. We had to wait for the medicine to work.

I tried to be brave, but I could not hold back my tears. I held her and spoke softly until I could tell she was reviving.

What I learned from this terrifying incident was to practice these emergency procedures frequently so that I would be better able to cope.

Sometimes diabetes gets overwhelming, but we count our blessings because we have each other for love and support. I know that our children will be able to run, laugh and do anything that other children can do. They just need to monitor their blood sugar levels, take their insulin, exercise and eat a well-balanced diet. Our entire family has begun to lead a healthier lifestyle.

I know in my heart that I am doing my best to educate my children about diabetes, letting them know that they can control their disease. Diabetes does not have to control them. Life can be wonderful, even after the devastating news.

I know there are times when you think you won't be able to get through the day, but somehow you do. You should be proud of yourself because caring for a child or children with diabetes is not easy. You are not alone. We are all going through basically the same difficulties. Try to find a support group near you or, if you can, find a family member who would be willing to help you through the tougher days.

Don't give up because the child has diabetes. As hard as this may be to believe, you will find that you will become much closer to the child. You will know this child so well. My husband and I cherish every new day that we have to share with our children. Our lives are much richer because of what we have been through and have handled together. I am truly blessed with such wonderful children.

My husband and my children are my greatest loves. We need to give our children a lot of love, patience and positive encouragement. You will feel wonderful when you see your children lovingly enjoying life in spite of their diabetes. Remember, with the right management of their diabetes, children can do anything they strive for. Nothing should stand in their way.

My life is now devoted to my children and family. They come first in every aspect of my life. To me, there is not a job on earth that is more important than raising children. What greater gift in life is there than giving children all the opportunities that life offers! Through the support of a loving, attentive family, success in life will not be diminished by diabetes.

God bless you. You are the reason I wrote this book. I pray this book will help and encourage you as a family to live each day to its fullest. Life has many beautiful things to offer and children have many things to share.

Treasure life.

2

About Diabetes

Diabetes mellitus

Diabetes mellitus is a disorder of the metabolism characterized by an abnormally high concentration of sugar in the blood. Most of the food we eat is broken down by the digestive juices into differ-ent substances, one of which is a simple sugar called glucose. After digestion, the glucose passes into the bloodstream, where it be-comes available for the body's cells to use for growth and energy. In order for the glucose to get into the cells, insulin must be present. Insulin is a hormone produced by the pancreas. Insulin acts like the key placed in a lock that opens the door for sugar to enter cells.

When people without diabetes eat, the pancreas automatically produces the right amount of insulin to handle the glucose. In children with diabetes, however, the pancreas produces either too little or no insulin at all, or the body's cells do not respond to the insulin that is produced. As a result, glucose builds up in the blood and overflows into the urine, where it is lost. Thus, the body loses a major source of fuel.

There are two major types of diabetes. Type 1, known as insulin-dependent diabetes mellitus (IDDM), is an autoimmune disease. My children have Type 1 diabetes. The pancreatic cells that produce insulin, called the beta cells, are destroyed by the body's own immune system. The pancreas then produces little or no insulin. To live, people with Type 1 diabetes require daily injections of insulin. At present, scientists do not know exactly what causes the body's immune system to attack the beta cells, but they believe that both genetic factors and environmental agents are involved. Type 1 accounts for 5 to 10 percent of the diagnosed cases of diabetes in the United States.

Type 1 develops most often in children or young adults, although the disorder can appear at any age. Symptoms of Type 1 usually develop over a short period of time (i.e., over two to four weeks), although beta cell destruction can begin months, or even years, earlier. Symptoms include increased thirst and urination. If diabetes is not diagnosed and properly treated with insulin, the person can lapse into a life-threatening coma called DKA (diabetic ketoacidosis). When sugar is unavailable to the body for use as fuel because of insulin deficiency, the body uses other energy sources. Fat is then broken down into a substance called "ketones." The ketones, like sugar, can spill over into the urine and accumulate in the bloodstream. When the ketone level is too high, a change in the blood chemistry called acidosis can result. This condition is life-threatening and requires immediate evaluation and treatment.

The most common form of diabetes is Type 2, or noninsulin-dependent diabetes mellitus (NIDDM). Ninety to 95 percent of people with diabetes have Type 2. This form of diabetes can develop in adults over the age of forty, although more children and younger adults are being diagnosed with it now. About 80 percent of people with Type 2 are overweight, have a sedentary lifestyle, are inactive and eat a high-fat, high-calorie diet, which contributes to the development of diabetes.

With Type 2 diabetes, the pancreas usually produces insulin, but for some reason, the body cannot use it effectively. The end result is the same as for Type 1 – an unhealthy build-up of glucose in the blood and an inability of the body to make efficient use of its main source of fuel.

The impact of diabetes

Diabetes is widely recognized as one of the leading causes of death and disability in the United States. In 1995, diabetes caused or contributed to more than 200,000 deaths. The true toll is probably much higher because diabetes was not listed on half of the death certificates of people who had diabetes. Diabetes is associated with long-term complications that affect almost every major organ of the body. Diabetes can cause blindness, heart disease, strokes or kidney failure, and can result in amputations or cause nerve damage and birth defects in babies born to women with diabetes. Fortunately, there have been advances in care and blood sugar monitoring. Instead of urine testing for glucose, for example, there are blood glucose monitors that have helped people achieve better glucose control and diminish the risk of complications.

In terms of medical care, treatment supplies, hospitalizations, time lost from work, disability payments, and premature death, diabetes cost this country over 100 billion dollars in 1997. Nearly one out of seven health care dollars is spent on diabetes and its complications.

Who has diabetes?

Almost everyone knows someone who has diabetes. Each year, 700,000 to 800,000 people are diagnosed with the disease. Approximately 16 million people in the United States have diabetes mellitus, a serious, lifelong disorder that is, as yet, incurable. More than a third of these people do not know they have diabetes and are not under medical care.

Although diabetes occurs often in older adults, it is one of the most common chronic disorders of children in the United States. Each year 10,000 to 15,000 children and teenagers in the U.S. are diagnosed with diabetes.

Diabetes can develop in people of any age or ethnic background, although some groups appear to be at higher risk for certain types of diabetes. Type 1 occurs equally between males and females, and it is more common in the white, non-Hispanic population. Some northern European countries, including Finland and Sweden, have very high rates of Type 1, with one in 200 children getting it before the age of 16. One out of 300 children in the United States will develop Type 1 diabetes, and over one in 500,000 people are insulin dependent.

Type 2 frequently occurs among African-Americans, Hispanics and Native Americans. Compared with non-Hispanic whites, diabetes rates are 60 percent higher in African-Americans and 110 to 120 percent higher in Mexican-Americans and Puerto Ricans. Native Americans have the highest rate of diabetes in the world. Among the Pima Indians, for example, half of all adults have Type 2 diabetes. The rate of diabetes is likely to increase because older people, Hispanics and other minorities make up the fastest growing portion of the U.S. population. Also, as the frequency of obesity in children and adults continues to rise in this country, the risk of developing Type 2 rises.

Children and diabetes

Doctors once believed that diabetes was inherited, but they now know that other factors play a role in who gets the disease. It seems that diabetes occurs in people with a genetic predisposition for diabetes who are exposed to viruses or other unknown agents in the environment. These factors set off the immune system, which damages the beta cells that make insulin in the pancreas. Damage is thought to arise from an autoimmune attack on the beta cells. It is the body's immune system—specifically lymphocytes—that attacks and kills one's own beta cells.

The destruction of the pancreas is not complete immediately. Some insulin-producing beta cells may remain for a few months or up to a year after diagnosis. During this time, the so-called "honeymoon," it may be easier to control the child's blood sugar level. Although excellent blood glucose levels are thought by some to prolong the honeymoon period, the time will come when all the beta cells are destroyed. Once gone, no insulin can be produced by the body, causing people with the disease to become "insulin dependent." All the insulin they require must be taken by injection each day.

If a child experiences any of the following symptoms, you need to consult a physician. The doctor or nurse will either prick a finger or draw some blood and test the blood sugar level. Also, they may test urine for ketones, which are the breakdown product of fat.

Symptoms

Often, the onset of diabetes is so rapid that the person has little warning—usually just a few days or weeks. Sometimes diabetes is hard to recognize because the symptoms are similar to those of the flu.

The most common symptoms are
- frequent urination (polyuria)
- extreme thirst and increased drinking (polydipsia)
- irritability – the person cries for no reason, is cranky, angry, demanding, or exhibits other out-of-character behavior
- weight loss
- fatigue – the person doesn't seem to want to do much, and appears weak
- sometimes, increased appetite (polyphagia) followed by loss of appetite
- nausea, vomiting
- infections such as a yeast infection in the vagina or boils on the skin
- frequent bladder infections
- blurred vision

3

Treatment of Diabetes

BEFORE THE DISCOVERY OF INSULIN in 1921, people with Type 1 diabetes died within a few years of the onset of the disease. Diabetes was called the "wasting disease" because, without insulin, the glucose from food could not be used as fuel. People gradually became thinner and thinner and eventually died. Although insulin is not considered a cure for diabetes, its discovery was the major breakthrough in diabetes treatment. Today, daily injections of insulin are the basic therapy for Type 1 diabetes. Insulin injections must be balanced with diet, exercise, and daily testing of blood glucose levels. Careful adjustments of the insulin dosage levels are made based on the level of sugar in the blood. Diet and exercise form the basis for management of Type 2. Achieving ideal weight loss is very important for obese Type 2 patients.

The goal of diabetes management is to keep blood glucose levels as close to the normal (nondiabetic) range as possible. Normal fasting blood glucose levels in nondiabetic individuals is 70-110mg/dl. A recent study, sponsored by the National Institute of Diabetes and Digestive and Kidney Diseases (NIDDK), has proven that keeping blood glucose levels near the normal range reduces the risk of developing major complications of diabetes. This nine-year study, called the Diabetes Control and Complications Trial (DCCT), was completed in June of 1992 and included 1,441 individuals with Type 1 diabetes (see Chapter 14). The DCCT compared two treatment approaches: conventional management, which mainly aimed to avoid extremely high or low blood glucose levels, and intensive management, which focused on keeping blood glucose levels as close to normal as possible. The purpose of the study was to determine whether intensive management of diabetes affects the development and severity of eye, kidney, and nerve complications of diabetes. The study findings showed that the people in the intensively managed group had significantly lower rates of complications. Researchers believe that the DCCT findings have important implications for the treatment of Type 2 as well as Type 1 diabetes.

People with diabetes must, however, avoid having blood glucose levels that are too low too frequently. This condition is known as hypoglycemia. When blood glucose levels drop too low, the person may become nervous and shaky, judgment may be impaired, and eventually, if left untreated, may have a seizure or lapse into an unconscious state (coma). The treatment for hypoglycemia is to eat or drink something with sugar in it, followed by foods containing complex carbohydrates and protein.

When blood glucose levels rise too high, a condition known as hyperglycemia occurs. A high glucose level can occur in people with either Type 1 or Type 2 diabetes. If allowed to continue to the extreme, both glucose abnormalities are potentially life-threatening.

Hyperglycemia

Hyperglycemia is a condition characterized by high blood glucose levels.

Hyperglycemia may develop slowly or rapidly. It may not become an emergency problem unless the glucose level exceeds 240 to 400 mg/dl and ketoacidosis develops. Untreated ketoacidosis is a serious problem.

These are a few reasons for hyperglycemia:

- too much food
- not enough exercise
- not enough insulin
- illness
- unusual stress

Many warning signs of hyperglycemia can develop slowly. Listen to the child when he or she tells you about

- extreme thirst, often with a dry or "cotton" mouth
- frequent urination
- nausea
- pain in the stomach
- feeling more sleepy than usual
- feeling more irritable
- blurry vision
- a bad headache

To prevent the child from getting hyperglycemia, first you should get the blood glucose back down to the correct level. Ideally, fasting blood sugars should be maintained between 80 and 120mg/dl. However, blood sugar goals vary with age and other factors. Young children who are at an increased risk of low blood sugar levels would be well controlled with fasting and blood glucose levels that are between 100–170.

Hyperglycemia can become a serious problem. In the short term, prolonged hyperglycemia can lead to dehydration. If the blood glucose stays too high over a long time—often years—it may cause serious complications. The DCCT has shown that long-term hyperglycemia causes eye, kidney and nerve damage which, if remedied early, can be reversed with improved blood sugar control.

The best way to control blood glucose levels is to
- eat the right amount of food (a dietitian can help you)

- participate in a daily exercise routine

- make sure the child is getting the right amount of insulin, and that the injection site is rotated

- monitor blood glucose before each meal. Sometimes a blood sugar test is necessary two hours after a meal and prior to bedtime.

If you follow these four steps, you will improve the child's blood glucose level dramatically. It is important to test blood sugar levels every day, not just when they are high. Remember that you are dealing with your child's life. Once you get into the proper routine you will find that it is not so difficult. You *can* do it.

Ketones

Ketones are formed from the breakdown of fats and are used by the muscles for energy. When there is not enough insulin in the body, ketones are overproduced. They will accumulate in the blood and eventually spill into the urine.

A child with diabetes can be diagnosed as having a high level of ketones if he or she fails to receive insulin for one day or longer. In this situation, ketoacidosis usually develops. This condition involves an accumulation of ketones in the blood and urine, producing deeper and more rapid breathing (called "Kussmaul" respiration). A gradual loss of consciousness may occur, especially in younger children with diabetes. If it is not treated promptly, the person becomes extremely ill and may die.

Ketoacidosis

Ketoacidosis occurs when a child does not have enough insulin to move the glucose into the cells for energy, and excessive fat breakdown occurs. When cells do not get the glucose they need, blood glucose levels go up, and the body starts to break down fat, which is converted into ketones. Although ketones can be used for energy by the body for a while, the rapid accumulation of ketones in blood changes the blood chemistry. Acidosis can result, leading to coma and, eventually, death.

Ketoacidosis can develop very quickly. During illness, especially when the child has a cold, infections, the flu, or the like, you should check the urine for the presence of ketones. You should also check for ketones when the blood glucose level is over 240mg/dl.

There are several symptoms that warn you when ketoacidosis is developing:
- extreme thirst
- frequent urination
- stomach pains or nausea
- vomiting
- weight loss
- "fruity" or "sweet" breath

Children should be tested for ketones
- when their blood glucose level is 240mg/dl or higher
- any time they are ill, regardless of the blood glucose level
- when they develop some warning symptoms of ketoacidosis

The easiest way to find out whether the child has ketones is by using ketone strips or tablets. All you do with a ketone strip is dip it into a sample of urine, then wait for fifteen seconds while it changes color. The timing is important because colors continue to change. Compare the color of the strip to a color chart on the bottle. If ketones are present, you need to record the level in a diabetes logbook. Be sure to tell the doctor or nurse so he or she can help you determine how much additional insulin the child will need.

Acetest tablets are an alternative to ketone strips. The tablets also cause a color change, which you compare to the chart on the bottle.

Whether you use strips or tablets, it is important to replace the cap on the bottle they come in. Accuracy can be affected by humidity, as well as the age of the strips or tablets.

When you know the child has ketones, have the child drink sugarless liquids, and call the doctor or nurse educator immediately. He or she will let you know whether the child should take more insulin, drink more fluids or go to the hospital. By speaking to the doctor or nurse in a timely fashion, hospitalization may not be necessary.

If ketoacidosis is not treated with insulin and intravenous fluids, three things will happen:
1. The blood glucose level will continue to climb.
2. The ketones will continue to build up in the blood, causing acidosis. Ketones appear in the urine before they become elevated in the bloodstream.
3. With severe acidosis and dehydration, heart failure, stroke and coma can develop. If left untreated, ketoacidosis is fatal.

If you cannot reach the doctor when the child is sick, take the child to the emergency room right away.

Hypoglycemia

Hypoglycemia occurs when the blood glucose level falls too low (below 60mg/dl). This condition is also called an "insulin reaction." It can happen very quickly.

Causes of hypoglycemia:
- The child doesn't eat enough food at mealtime or misses a snack.
- Excessive exercise.
- Too much insulin is given.

Symptoms of hypoglycemia:
- shaky hands and legs
- dizziness
- headache
- irritability
- heart beats faster
- confusion
- lips may tingle and feel numb
- stomach hurts
- personality change. The child may react and seem out of control, or a normally outgoing person may become withdrawn
- crying all the time for no reason

An untreated low blood sugar level can result in seizures, coma or even death if it is not treated quickly. A low blood sugar condition can usually be treated by drinking something with sugar in it, like juice or regular soda, or by taking glucose tablets. You should always carry a snack such as juice, hard sugar candy, peanut butter crackers, cake frosting in a tube or glucose tablets. Make sure the food is appropriate for the age of the child. Small hard candies, for example, can pose a choking hazard to toddlers.

My children experience hypoglycemia often because I try to keep their sugar levels as close to normal as possible—in the 80-160mg/dl range—but sometimes it's difficult. Children's daily routines or eating patterns often vary. If the children do not eat the correct amount of carbohydrates or exercise more than anticipated, their blood sugar levels can drop lower than anticipated.

It is mentally draining for me when my children have hypoglycemia. There have been times when my daughter has fallen on the floor, kicking her feet and crying, "Mommy, hurry, my legs are shaking; they're going to fall off." As a parent, you move as fast and efficiently as you can, but sometimes it feels like an eternity before the symptoms abate. I respond immediately by giving her 4 ounces of orange juice, and then I measure her sugar level to see how low she is. I follow up with protein and carbohydrates according to her blood sugar reading. Sometimes after I have given her the correct amount of juice and food, Jennifer tells me that her legs still are shaking. I explain to her that it takes about 15 to 30 minutes to feel better. When this happens I rock her or read to her until she feels better. This has happened to her most often after she has come in from playing hard outside. I not only treat the medical emergencies, but I console and comfort during these difficult times.

I try to estimate how much exercise my children will be doing each day. If I can figure it out, I usually give them less H (Humalog insulin) or give them a larger snack (more carbohydrates) to sustain them for the amount of exercise they will be doing.

Foot Care

Children and adults with diabetes are at a greater risk of amputation of their toes, feet and legs. Amputation is 15 times more common among people with diabetes. Each year, more than 56,000 amputations are performed on people with diabetes.

It is extremely important to keep blood sugar levels as close to normal as possible and to follow a few simple rules to help reduce the risk of any type of foot problem.

1. Keep feet clean and make sure they are completely dry after washing, especially between toes.
2. If feet are dry, apply a small amount of lotion to them after the bath or swimming. Rub it in well so that the feet are not left damp. You can also use foot powder if feet perspire. (Do not apply lotion between the toes.)
3. Keep toenails trimmed. Cut them by following the contour of the nails. If a corner of a nail is sharp, file it down until it is smooth.
4. If there is an ingrown toenail and it becomes red and

sore, call your physician immediately.

5. Check feet on a daily basis for cuts, blisters or scratches. Also, check between the toes for cracks.

6. Never cut any corns or calluses off.

7. Never walk barefoot on hot surfaces.

8. In the winter, wear extra-warm socks and shoes to protect feet from the cold.

9. Check the insides of shoes to make sure that there are no torn linings or any rough areas at all. Wear well-fitting and comfortable shoes at all times. Shoes that are too tight can cause blisters and other problems with feet. Keep all shoes clean and dry to reduce the chance for fungus to grow. Shoes that are too narrow or pointy can cause corns, calluses and blisters.

10. Make sure your physician examines the child's feet at every visit.

4

Testing and Injecting

OTHER THAN YOUNG CHILDREN, people with diabetes are usually responsible for their own day-to-day care. However, children with diabetes can manage age-appropriate tasks. They should also be under the general care of a doctor who monitors their diabetes control and checks for diabetes complications. Doctors who specialize in diabetes are called endocrinologists or diabetologists.

In addition, people with diabetes often see other specialists such as ophthalmologists for an eye examination, podiatrists for foot care, dietitians for meal-planning guidance, and diabetes educators for instruction in day-to-day care. Also, it may be necessary to consult a counselor at some point for emotional support, as diabetes 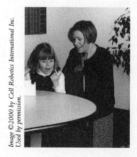 can be difficult for children to handle, particularly in the adolescent years. Or, if the stress of day-to-day living seems monumental, it may be helpful to talk with a caring person who just listens and offers suggestions, such as a psychologist, psychiatrist, social worker, clergy member or another parent of a child with diabetes.

Testing blood sugar

Blood glucose testing is the most important part of your child's diabetes management routine because it allows you to know exactly what your child's levels are at any time. Depending on the individual treatment plan spelled out by your diabetes health care team, the blood sugar level should be checked prior to injecting insulin, as well as before breakfast, lunch, dinner and bedtime, plus whenever the child is ill or acting out of character. You can balance the blood sugar with exercise, food and insulin if you know what the blood sugar level is. The knowledge of the child's levels allows you and your doctor, dietitian, or educator to make the needed changes.

Testing Procedure

To check the sugar level with a glucose meter, you will need the meter, test strips, a lancing device (also known as a "finger pricker"—usually, one comes with the meter kit), lancets, a cotton ball and sometimes an alcohol swab.

1. Before testing, the child should wash his or her hands with soap and warm water. The warm water is important because it stimulates blood flow to the fingers. After drying hands thoroughly, have the child hang the hand down for about 10 seconds before pricking the finger. If it is not possible to wash the child's hands, then wipe the finger with an alcohol swab, and wait a few seconds for the alcohol to dry.

2. Turn the meter on and insert the test strip when the meter indicates.

3. To avoid soreness, choose a site on the side of the fingertip, not directly on the top of the pad. The top of the fingertips is very sensitive and should not be used. Also, rotate the finger sites each time you test to avoid the formation of calluses.

4. Hold the pricker firmly against the side of the finger and press the button. If you are using a laser device, insert finger into the opening and press the button.

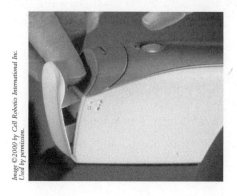

Image ©2000 by Cell Robotics International Inc. Used by permission.

Hold the hand down for a couple of seconds. To get a good size drop of blood, "milk" the finger by rubbing it down, away from the hand.

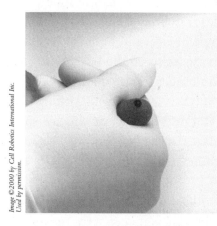

Image ©2000 by Cell Robotics International Inc. Used by permission.

Turn the finger over so that the drop of blood can be placed on the test strip until the meter begins to count down. (This procedure varies slightly depending on what type of meter you have). Place a cotton ball on the finger and hold for a few seconds to help stop the bleeding. Wait for a few seconds for the test result to appear on the meter. Record your results in a logbook.

Be sure to follow the specific instructions for your particular blood drawing and testing devices. The procedures you need to follow may vary slightly, especially if you are using a different kind of tester or pricker, such as one that works with a laser rather than a lancet.

Injecting insulin

Insulin must be injected rather than taken in pill form because stomach acids destroy insulin that is taken orally before it can start to work. Scientists are looking for new ways to administer insulin, but injections into the skin are the only technique that exists at present.

It is important to prepare your syringe correctly so that the insulin can work in the child's body properly. When you are instructed by your physician to use two or three types of insulin, they can be mixed into the same syringe so that you give all the insulin in one injection at a time, rather than in multiple injections.

One type of clear insulin is called Regular, which is a fast-acting insulin. Another type of clear insulin is called Humalog fast-acting insulin, which starts working in the body in about fifteen minutes to decrease the blood sugar levels rapidly.

An additional kind of insulin is NPH long-acting insulin, and it always appears cloudy. However, if you see small floating stars, particles, or snowflakes in the NPH bottle, discard it. The presence of these particles indicates that the NPH insulin is old and will not work efficiently.

The drug manufacturers recommend that once you have opened a bottle of insulin, you keep it for only a month before discarding it.

In the morning, I used to give my children Regular and NPH insulin. Now that Humalog is available, I give them only Humalog and NPH insulin. The reason for this change is so that they do not have so many hypoglycemic reactions. Also, Humalog stays in the body for only about 2½ hours, so this insulin does not affect their morning snack, whereas Regular insulin did.

Keep in mind that when you are mixing insulins, they need to be drawn up in a specific order: CLEAR BEFORE CLOUDY. You need to draw up the clear (Regular) and/or clear (Humalog) insulin into the syringe first, and then draw up the cloudy (NPH) insulin.

If you draw up the cloudy insulin first, before drawing up the clear insulin, you run the risk of contaminating the clear insulin. If this were to happen, the regular insulin would work during its appropriate time. But hours later, you would have additional NPH insulin acting to lower the blood sugar in an unplanned way.

Take your time in drawing up the correct amount of insulin. If you have any doubts about what you have done, it is best to discard the syringe or the insulin in the syringe and start over.

Preparing the syringe

The supplies that you will need are alcohol swabs, a syringe and the bottle(s) of insulin.

1. Wash your hands well.

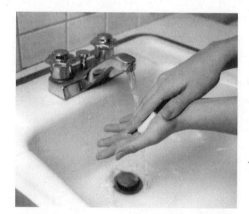

2. Gently ROLL (DO NOT shake) the bottle between the palms of your hands at least twenty times to mix the solution evenly. This step is extremely important because if the insulin is not mixed well, you may not inject the proper concentration of insulin, which can result in blood sugar levels that are either too low or too high.

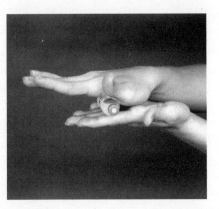

• • • NEVER SHAKE A BOTTLE OF INSULIN • • •

3. Pull the plunger of the syringe down to let in the required number of units of air. The units of air correspond to the TOTAL units of insulin that you need to inject. Example: if you will inject two units of Humalog insulin and four units of NPH insulin, then you will draw a total of six units of air into the syringe.

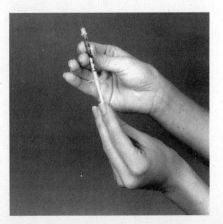

4. Wipe the top of the insulin bottle with an alcohol swab to disinfect it where the syringe needle enters, and wait a few moments for it to dry.

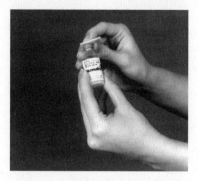

5. Push the syringe needle through the top of the insulin bottle.

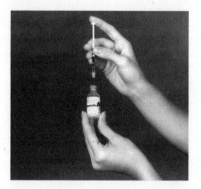

6. Push the air into the insulin bottle by depressing the plunger. Leave the needle in the bottle to make it easier for you to draw out the insulin.

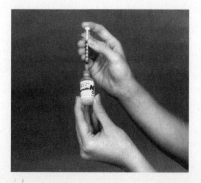

7. Turn your insulin bottle and syringe upside down. Hold the insulin bottle and needle with one hand.

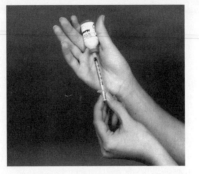

8. With the other hand, slowly pull the plunger out until the correct number of units of insulin fills the syringe. If you get too much insulin in the syringe, depress the plunger until you see the correct number of units.

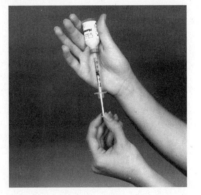

Examine your syringe for any air bubbles. The presence of an air bubble prevents the correct amount of insulin from being drawn up. If you see any air bubbles, push the insulin back into the bottle and repeat step eight. If there are no bubbles, then you can remove the needle from the insulin bottle.

If you are using two or more types of insulin, repeat steps four through eight with each bottle, being scrupulously careful to draw up the cloudy insulin LAST. Remember, the rule is CLEAR BE-FORE CLOUDY.

· · · REMEMBER, CLEAR BEFORE CLOUDY · · ·

Giving the injection

The first thing I was taught by the diabetes education team was how to give an insulin injection. It was extremely difficult for me to inflict pain on my baby. He did not understand what was happening. He was so frightened. Since then, I began holding him for a little while before and after an injection. I want him to know that I love him very much. It hurts me much more mentally to give the injection than he suffers physically from the needle.

Giving injections gets easier with time. Both of my children tolerate their injections well now. They let me know where their next injection spot should be, since we rotate the injections among arms, legs and buttocks. I still hug them before and after an injection because sometimes it really does hurt. At times I hit a blood vessel and we see a tiny drop of blood, or a small bruise mark occurs. I feel so bad when this happens, but they know I do the best I can.

By giving an injection the right way, it doesn't hurt much, and sometimes it doesn't hurt at all. When I first started to give my son Joseph his insulin, he was only 21 months old. Injection times were frustrating and difficult. My husband, Joe, was rarely home, but when he was, there was always some excuse why he could not give Joseph the injection.

Joseph hated any kind of shot. He would kick, roll around and scream the minute he saw the syringe. So I had to figure out a way to minimize the trauma for him and myself. Many times I would cry before I even gave him his injection, because I felt that I was hurting my wonderful baby. I feared that he would grow up to hate me. But that isn't the case. The older Joseph is, the more he has come to understand why I must give him these injections. We have a special bond now, and I know he loves me even more.

There is more than one way to keep the child still enough to administer the injections. You may find that your own method works best for you, or you can try a couple of ways that have been successful for me.

Example 1 (works well for children up to 7 years):

1. Wash your hands well. Prepare the syringe with the correct amount of insulin.

2. Take the syringe to a room where there is a chair that you can sit in to give the child the injection. Place the syringe near the chair.

3. Sit the child on your lap. I cuddle with my children for a few seconds first.

4. When you are ready, place the child's legs between your thighs. Cross one of your legs over his knees.

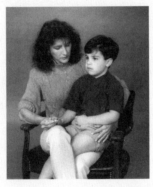

5. Next, lean him to one side on your lap. Put your arm across his chest in front of his body.

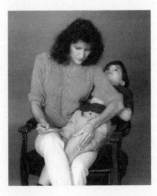

6. Once he is secure and still, remove the cap from the syringe, either with your hand or with your teeth.

7. Clean the injection site on the child's body with an alcohol swab. Wait a moment for the alcohol to dry.

8. At the injection site, pinch some skin between your thumb and fingers. Push the needle through the skin. Depress the plunger all the way down to force the insulin into the body. Remove the needle from the skin. Place a finger over the injected spot for a few seconds.

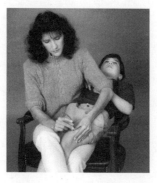

Example 2:

1. Wash your hands well. Prepare the syringe with the correct amount of insulin.

2. Go to a room where there is a couch, bed or changing table. Place the syringe nearby, so you can reach it when you have the child in place.

3. Lay the child down on the couch, bed or changing table.

4. Lie across the child's body, securing the child's legs and arms.

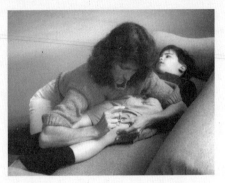

5. Once he is secure and still, remove the cap from the syringe.

6. Clean the injection site on the child's body with an alcohol swab. Wait a moment for the alcohol to dry.

8. At the injection site, pinch some skin between your thumb and fingers. Push the needle through the skin. Depress the plunger all the way down to force the insulin into the body. Remove the needle from the skin. Place a finger over the injected spot for a few seconds.

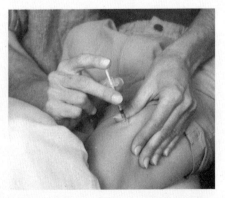

When I finished giving my son his injections, he would cry. I would hold him immediately and let him know how much I loved him. Trying to be strong in front of him was difficult, because many times I just couldn't hold back the tears. I knew he was afraid of needles and that they were sometimes painful.

But within four months, Joseph did not seem to mind getting his injections. Now he will let me give him his injection anywhere I want, except in his belly. The reason he doesn't like that spot is that he's convinced we will inject the insulin into his food! Joseph now knows that he has to have an injection in the morning and in the evening. He knows that if he does not take his insulin, he will become extremely ill and eventually die.

From time to time when you are giving an injection, you might hit a blood vessel and it will hurt or sting. There is nothing you can do but be sympathetic to the child. Understand that you did your best. It is not your fault. Remember, you need to give them a lot of love, understanding and, most of all, patience.

Read to your children about diabetes or, if they can read, give them articles and books on the subject. It is my belief that the more information you give them, the easier it is for them to deal with the disease.

The glucagon emergency kit

If the child passes out, cannot swallow or goes into a seizure, then you need to use glucagon. This medicine raises the blood sugar level quickly by releasing stored glucose (glycogen). You inject glucagon into any fatty tissue that you can reach, then call the doctor immediately to let him or her know what is happening. It is important that you know where the glucagon is located at all times. You may need more than one glucagon kit. If possible, keep one in your diabetes carrying case as well, just in case you are outside the home when hypoglycemia occurs.

Within five to 15 minutes, the child should respond to the glucagon. If not, call the doctor immediately to let him or her know what is going on.

Often people vomit or feel sick to their stomach after receiving glucagon. Sips of sugared soda without the fizz or Gatorade may help. To quickly eliminate the "fizz" or carbonation from soda pop, add a few tablespoons of warm to hot water to release the gas bubbles. Don't add too much water or you may over-dilute the soda.

We purchased three glucagon emergency kits and placed one of them in the kitchen and one in each of the children's carrying cases. Everyone in our family and our caregivers know where the glucagon kits are located in case of an emergency. As with any medication, make sure the adults or mature caregivers have access to the glucagon. Keep the medicine away from small children.

I thank God that in the eight years since my children developed diabetes, I have only had to use the glucagon once (and once is enough for me). I believe it is because I monitor the children so closely. Even in the middle of the night, sometimes I feel that I should check their sugar levels if their activity has been heavy or food intake has been less than normal for them. There have been many times when their levels were very low. When this happens, I quickly give them 4 ounces of juice and a few crackers with cheese or peanut butter.

When my children feel poorly, I try to take their blood glucose levels first and treat them accordingly. If they have symptoms and I cannot check their levels, I start treating them immediately with some juice. While they are drinking the juice, I take their blood glucose levels.

If my children's levels are 60 to 70mg/dl, I give them 1 to 4 ounces of juice or some food. If the levels are 49 or below, I give them 4 ounces of juice, one glucose tablet and a snack.

It is better to raise their blood glucose a little too high than to let it get too low. With time, you will know how much food or juice is needed to raise the child's blood sugar to a higher range.

Injecting glucagon

1. Remove the bottle and glucagon from the case.
    Remove the flip-top seal from the bottle.

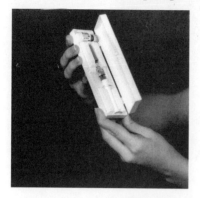 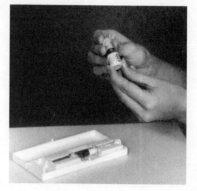

2. Remove the needle protector from the syringe.

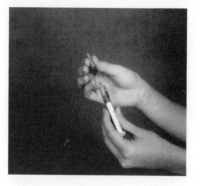

3. Inject the entire amount of liquid in the syringe into
    the bottle of glucagon.

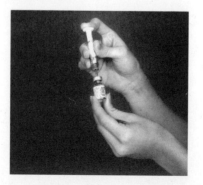

4. Remove the syringe from the bottle.

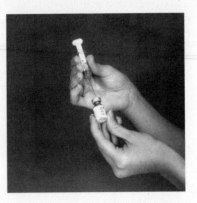

5. Shake the bottle from side to side gently until the solution becomes clear. (If it is not clear, do not use the glucagon.)

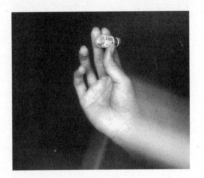

6. Using the same syringe, withdraw the correct amount of medicine for an emergency as directed by your doctor.

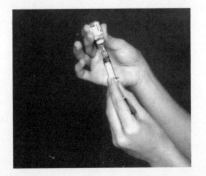

7. Inject the glucagon as you would insulin. Apply some light pressure at the injection site and withdraw the needle. But if the child is having a seizure, it will be difficult to keep the child still. Inject the medicine into any fatty tissue that you can reach safely.

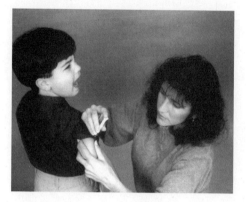

8. If the child is lying down, turn the child on his or her side. Quite often, children who have received glucagon will vomit after they become conscious. By turning them onto their sides, any emesis (vomit, food or liquid substance) will drain out and not get into their lungs.

9. Once the child becomes responsive after a glucagon injection, you need to give him or her sugar from some fast-acting source, such as orange or other fruit juice. Next, give the child some cheese or peanut butter crackers. A well-balanced snack containing protein and carbohydrates will help maintain blood sugar levels.

10. Call the doctor to report that the child had an episode of low blood sugar (hypoglycemia or an insulin reaction).

NOTE: *If you have any doubts at all, call for emergency assistance.*

5

Supplies for Diabetes Management

When our son was diagnosed with diabetes, we were given some guidance by our nurse educator regarding the kind of supplies we needed to make our lives easier. Often, rebate incentives are given toward the purchase of the meters, so it pays to ask before you buy. Below is some information on various meters, visual glucose strips and other supplies to help manage diabetes.

Blood Glucose Meters

Most blood glucose meters can be purchased at the pharmacy. Often, rebate incentives are given toward the purchase price of the meters, so it pays to ask before you buy. Some of the more popular meters are listed below along with manufacturers' contact information.

Accu-Chek Complete, Advantage, Simplicity and Instant
(Roche Diagnostics)
1-800-858-8072
www.accu-chek.com

AtLast Blood Glucose System
(Amira Medical)
1-877-264-7263
www.amiramed.com

Exac Tech
(Abbott Laboratories, MediSense Products)
1-800-537-3575
www.diabetesnow.com

Fast Take, One Touch BASIC, One Touch Profile and Sure Step
(Lifescan Inc.)
1-800-227-8862 (U.S)
1-800-663-5521 (Canada)
www.lifescan.com

Glucometer Dex, Elite and Elite XL
(Bayer Corporation)
1-800-348-8100 (U.S.)
1-800-268-7200 (Canada)
www.glucometerdex.com

In Charge Diabetes System
(LXN Corporation)
1-877-596-8379
www.inchargenow.com

Precision Q.I.D. and Precision Xtra
(Abbott Laboratories, MediSense Products)
1-800-527-3339
www.medisense.com

Prestige LX
(Home Diagnostics Inc.)
1-800-342-7226
www.prestigesmartsystem.com

Visual glucose test strips

Visual glucose test strips do not require any meters. Each test strip works in a slightly different manner. Be sure to read the directions before using them. Details are given here for some test strips.

Chemstrip bG : (Roche Diagnostic)
Color chart increments (mg/dl):
    20, 40, 80, 120, 180, 240, 400, 800
Instructions: Apply blood to test area; wipe after 1 minute; read after 2 minutes.

Glucostix Reagent Strips • (Bayer Corporation)
Color chart increments (mg/dl):
    20, 40, 70, 110, 140, 180, 250, 400, 800
Instructions: Apply blood to test area; blot after 30 seconds; wait an additional 90 seconds; read.

Supreme Strips • (Chronimed)
Color chart increments (mg/dl):
    low, 20, 40, 70, 120, 180, 240, 400, high
Instructions: Apply blood to test area; wait 60 seconds and turn strip over; compare color of reverse side to color chart.

Supplies

Lancet Devices

Lancet devices are usually provided as part of the blood glucose test kits. It's a great idea to keep a lancing device at home, at work or at school. They are not expensive and last a long time. You can purchase several different kinds at your local pharmacy.

Syringes

Some syringe needles are shorter and finer than others. A special coating on the needle acts as a lubricant, which makes the injection less painful. Syringes are available in ³⁄₁₀-cc, ½-cc and 1-cc. Determining what cc's to use will depend on how many units are given in the injection.

Insulin

Types of insulin: Lispro (Humalog), Humulin Regular, Humulin NPH, Lente, and Ultralente. The most commonly used strength of insulin in the United States is 100 units per ml. Insulin is available only by prescription.

Glucagon Emergency Kit

The glucagon kit for severe hypoglycemia (low blood glucose level) consists of a syringe filled with diluting solution and one bottle of glucagon. If my son cannot eat or swallow anything because of a severe blood sugar low, I will use the glucagon. For emergencies, we carry a glucagon kit in our diabetes carrying case and have a couple of kits in our home. Glucagon kits are available only by prescription.

Frosting in a Tube

Frosting in a tube for emergency is great to have on hand. If the child does not want to eat or drink, you can squeeze some frosting in the side of their mouth. This weill help raise the blood glucose level. You can easily carry a couple of tubes in the diabetes carrying case, glove box, purse, or even in your pocket. The frosting comes in several different colors. You may prefer to use white frosting instead of the colored frosting because it may stain the mouth for a short time.

Glucose Tablets

These tablets are for insulin reactions. You can purchase them at most pharmacies. They come in lemon, orange, raspberry and grape flavors.

Alcohol Swabs
These swabs are used for cleaning the injection spot. You can purchase them at most drug stores.

Ketone Strips
These strips are used for testing ketones. When your child's glucose is 240mg or higher or the child is sick, you will need to check for ketones. You can purchase them at your local pharmacies.

100% Juice Box or 8.45-oz Gatorade Box Drink
We use 4-oz. juice box or Gatorade box when their blood sugar levels are too low. There are 15 to 17 grams of carbohydrates in each box. The boxes fit well in the carrying cases.

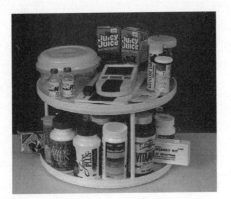

Lazy Susan
We have our lazy Susan on our kitchen counter. The supplies we keep on it are a meter, penlet, lancets, glucagon, glucose tablets, insulin, test strips, juices, self-care diary, glucose gel, peanut butter crackers and vitamins.

This picture shows how we have our lazy Susan set up.

REMEMBER: If you have smaller children in your household, you may need to place your supplies in an accessible place that is out of reach of the youngest ones.

Self-Care Diary

This is a small book that we use daily to keep track of blood sugar levels and insulin dosages. It is so important to keep good records of blood sugar levels, ketones and different foods or activities done on a particular day. This book will help you and your doctor to understand how blood sugar levels are fluctuating.

Carrying cases

There are different kinds of cases available for carrying your diabetes supplies. Each one comes in handy for various activities. Listed below are a few carrying cases that will carry diabetic supplies for your everyday needs.

Diabetic Carry-All
(Apothecary Products)
This case holds 2 vials of insulin, up to 6 syringes, alcohol swabs and I.D Card. This case is an all-nylon soft-side case with Velcro closure.

Dia-Pak Deluxe
(Medicool Inc.)
1-800-433-2469
This is a compact carrying case made of water-resistant nylon. It holds 2 vials of insulin, syringes, alcohol swabs, lancets, test strips, all blood glucose meters, and I.D. card. There is an optional shoulder strap or waist belt available for this case. It comes in different colors, too.

Medicool Protect All
(Medicool Inc.)
1-800-433-2469
Protect All keeps your insulin safely cool for up to twelve hours. The cooler holds your syringes, meter, test strips, lancing device,

lancets and alcohol swabs. It goes around the waist or over the shoulder.

Note: There are many other cases available. See your local pharmacy.

Medical ID

It is a good idea for a diabetic child to wear medical identification at all times. In case of an emergency, these tags provide information about the child's condition. The child might become disoriented, suffer a seizure or experience some other difficulty when no adults who are aware of the diabetes are around. If an emergency occurs, it is important that whoever is assisting the child is aware of the diabetes. If the child gets hurt at school and has to be taken to the hospital, the medical ID will let emergency room personnel know about the disease so that they do not attempt to administer a glucose IV, for example.

Medical IDs come in a variety of shapes, sizes, colors and forms, such as bracelets, necklaces, pendants or charms. The best kind of ID depends on the child's age and preferences. Naturally, you wouldn't want to put a necklace on a baby or toddler, but some kids like wearing a MediCharms Teddy Bear or Bunny Rabbit that has "Diabetes—Insulin" stamped on it. On the other hand, many older kids get a kick out of wearing colorful nylon bracelets, such as the ones from Safety Sport ID Inc., that feature an insert on which the diagnosis can be written.

There are several sources for medical IDs, including the local drugstore. A number of companies also display their wares on the Internet or take phone orders for home delivery.

American Medical Identifications Inc.
P.O. Box 925512
Houston, TX 77292
800/363-5985
713/695-0284
www.americanmedical-id.com

Beverly Hills Collar Co.
34611 Camino Capistrano
Capistrano Beach, CA 92624
800/891-2663
949/240-3825
www.kids-ID.com

Goldware
P.O. Box 22335
San Diego, CA 92192
800/669-7311
858/453-4005
www.medical-id.net

Life Alert
P.O. Box 386
Lynden, WA 98264
888/543-3253
www.tinman.com/life

Medic Alert Foundation U.S.
P.O. Box 1009
Turlock, CA 95381-9009
800/432-5378
209/668-3333
www.medicalert.org

Medic Assist
P.O. Box 117627
Carrollton, TX 75011
877/902-8969
214/902-8969
www.medicassist.com

Medical-ID.com
P.O. Box 50
Verbank, NY 12585
800/830-0546
www.medical-id.com

MediCharms
P.O. Box 558
Bryant, AR 72089
888/417-7591
501/847-5587
www.missbrooke.com

Safety Sport ID Inc.
4546 Rutherford Drive
Marietta, GA 30062
770/650-0091
www.safetysportid.com

Insulin Pen

For people who are on the go or are intimidated by the looks of a syringe, the insulin pen is great. The pen looks like an old-fashioned cartridge pen in your pocket. The pen has a needle and a cartridge of insulin in it.

There is no refrigeration needed after the first use. The pen is accurate and a convenient way to administer insulin. Below is a list of some of the manufacturers' contact list.

Autopen
(Owen Mumford, Inc.)
1-800-421-6936
www.owenmumford.com

BD Pen and BD Pen Mini
(BD)
1-888-232-2737
www.bd.com

Disetronic Pen
(Disetronic Medical Systems, Inc.)
1-800-280-7801
www.disetronic-usa.com

Humalog Mix 75-25, Humalog Pen, Humulin 70/30 Pen, and Humulin NPH Pen
(Eli Lilly and Company)
1-800-545-5979
www.lilly.com

NovoPen 3
(NovoNordisk)
1-800-727-6500
www.novonordisk-us.com

6

At School

IT IS ESSENTIAL FOR PARENTS to take their time to educate the teachers, coaches, aides, principals and other adults who will interact with the diabetic child regarding diabetes and the special care their child will need. The adults all need to know how to respond to an emergency situation and what steps to take when a child has an insulin reaction (low blood sugar). In addition, it is important for the child's classmates to gain some understanding of the disease so that the diabetic child can enjoy a normal school experience.

Sometimes an entire administration or school district must be introduced to the concept of diabetes and the care the diabetic child requires. There are federal laws protecting diabetic children that the school may not be aware of. Therefore, it is important that parents become familiar with these regulations so that they can ensure that their child is treated fairly and in accordance with the laws.

Educating teachers and staff

When our children were diagnosed with diabetes, the thought of their being away from home most of the day was frightening. We live 22 miles from the school, and no other children in the school have diabetes. Each year, we take the time to let the school staff know about diabetes.

It is extremely important that teachers and other staff members become familiar with the symptoms of low blood sugar, which is the most common medical emergency for a diabetic child. There are many causes for low blood sugar, including a day when the child hasn't eaten enough, has forgotten to eat his or her snack, or has exercised more then usual. The child's blood sugar level could also become low if he or she is taking too much insulin.

If the children feel poorly, they notify their teacher and immediately check their own blood sugar level. If they are too weak, the teacher will assist them.

My husband and I wear a pager at all times and carry a mobile phone with us. If the school needs us, we can be reached at any time.

This is what I did to educate the teachers and staff:

1. I gathered up all the brochures and articles that I could find on diabetes for the teachers to read.

2. I made an appointment with the teachers and staff. All the teachers came to the meeting and learned about diabetes and the type of supervision our children would need.

3. I put together an emergency kit for the children's classroom. The emergency kit stays right by the teacher's desk. The kit consists of a meter with penlet, lancets, meter strips, one glucagon kit, glucose tablets, two tubes of white frosting mix, one small pack of facial tissues,

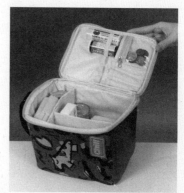

ketone strips, alcohol swabs, two packs of peanut butter crackers and two 4-oz. juices. This picture shows the cooler I use and the supplies.

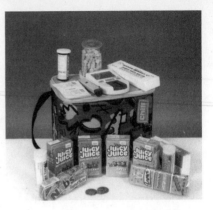

4. I explained to the teacher the importance of a quick response to a low blood sugar level.

5. I pricked my finger first to show them how it is done. Then they practiced on themselves and on each other.

6. We went over the steps they would need to take if the children were to have a seizure or lapse into an unconscious state. Then I explained how to administer glucagon.

7. I gave them a handout with the symptoms of low blood sugar. The sheet I use follows. I also let them know how low blood sugar affects my children specifically. Jennifer will act differently when her blood sugar level drops. She will cry, get upset and quite moody for no reason. Joseph, on the other hand, gets a little fidgety. If this occurs, the teacher needs to check their blood sugar levels. Each child is different, so let the teacher know how your child acts when his or her blood sugar level is low.

8. I made up an instruction sheet detailing how to treat their low blood sugar. An example of the teacher's instruction sheet follows. Every child with diabetes has different needs and responds differently when their blood sugar levels are low. You can make up your own instruction sheet or use the one shown here.

Symptoms of low blood sugar

- Weak, tired, shaky, hungry
- Headache
- Irritable
- Crying for no reason
- Dizziness
- Blurred vision
- Cannot concentrate
- Confused
- Personality changes, out of character

Teacher's instruction sheet

Child's Name _____

Mother's Phone # _____

Beeper # _____

Father's Phone # _____

Beeper # _____

Physician's Name _____

Physician's # _____

Time Blood Sugar
Is Taken _____

Blood Sugar Reading _____

Time _____

Ketones Yes _____ No _____

Special instructions

• • • **Always treat right away if their blood sugar is low** • • •

Extremely Low
If their blood glucose is 40 or below
Treat with   1 4-oz. Juice or 1 8-oz. Gatorade box drink
              2 glucose tablets
              2 peanut butter crackers

Low
If their blood glucose is 41 to 55
Treat with   1 4-oz. juice or 1 8-oz. Gatorade box drink
              1 glucose tablet
              2 peanut butter crackers

Moderately Low
If their blood glucose is 56 to 69
Treat with   1 4-oz. juice or 1 8-oz. Gatorade box drink
              1 peanut butter cracker

NOTE: It is a good idea to follow up with a blood glucose test 20-30 minutes later if the child is still feeling bad.

When their blood sugar is too low (less than 70) treat them, then call the parents immediately.

When their blood sugar is too high (greater than 240) check for ketones and call parents if there is more than a trace.

Educating classmates

We felt that not only did we need to educate the school staff, but also the children's classmates. The children needed to know the truth and as much as possible about diabetes. We didn't want Jennifer and Joseph to ever feel that they should have to hide from their disease.

On the first day of school, the children and I had a special diabetes education day for their classmates. This is what we did in their classroom:

1. We showed them a picture of a pancreas and explained how it works in the body.

2. We explained to them that diabetes is not something you can get from touching them.

3. We let everyone see and touch the supplies that are in the emergency kit.

4. Jennifer and Joseph let me prick their fingers in front of the students to see how it worked. The teachers then pricked themselves to show them not to be afraid.

5. We answered all of their questions: "Why do they have diabetes?" "Can they die from it?" "Can we catch it?"

6. We explained to the children why Jennifer and Joseph should not eat sugared candy. Then I gave all the children a small bag of sugar-free candy. They loved it!

The children were wonderful. Jennifer and Joseph do everything the other children do. Everyone is kind to them and no one makes them feel any different.

It sounds like a lot to do, but it is really not that much. If you would like some help in educating those at the school, ask your nurse educator to do it with you or for you. Most of them would be more than happy to help. Also, your nurse or doctor may have some handouts with information about diabetes that may be helpful to use.

After about three months we started to feel more comfortable with Jennifer's going to school. By the end of kindergarten she was testing her blood sugar level by herself. Joseph began testing his own blood sugar level in the first few months of kindergarten. Both of the children are handling their diabetes well.

Your child will be testing his or her own blood sugar level before you know it and will be able to tell the teacher that he or she is not feeling well. You will be so proud.

Party days at school

When there is a party, I volunteer to make cupcakes with sugar-free pudding for the icing. Also, a great party snack for the kids is Pudding Cream Puffs. (See page 148).

If there is a birthday party and they are having cake, I let my children have a piece of cake with some of the icing taken off. We want the children to participate just as the other kids do.

I provide sugar-free Kool-Aid or Crystal Light for the class to drink. For ice cream we provide Breyers No-Sugar-Added Vanilla, Chocolate or Strawberry. Other no-sugar-added, low-fat yogurts and ice creams are also available.

YOUR SCHOOL AND YOUR RIGHTS: PROTECTING CHILDREN WITH DIABETES AGAINST DISCRIMINATION IN SCHOOLS AND DAY CARE CENTERS [*]

Children with diabetes sometimes face problems in obtaining the care they need in schools and day care centers. [The following information] will help you understand the rights of children with diabetes and what you can do to make sure your child receives fair treatment.

[*] "Your School and Your Rights" copyright 1996 by the American Diabetes Association. Reprinted by permission.

The Laws

Students with disabilities have a right to a "free, appropriate public education" without discrimination. In addition, children in many private schools and day care centers are protected against discrimination on the basis of disability. These rights are guaranteed by the following federal civil rights and education laws:

Section 504 of the Rehabilitation Act of 1973

Section 504 protects individuals with disabilities against discrimination in any program or activity receiving federal financial assistance. This includes all public schools and day care centers and those private schools and centers that receive federal funds. To qualify for protection under Section 504, a child must have a physical or mental impairment that substantially limits one or more major life activities (such as learning), have a record of such an impairment, or be regarded as having such an impairment. Parents of qualifying children have the right to develop a Section 504 plan with their child's school. Schools can lose federal funding if they do not comply with this law.

The Americans with Disabilities Act

The Americans with Disabilities Act prohibits all schools and day care centers, except those run by religious organizations, from discriminating against children with disabilities. The standard for coverage is the same as under Section 504.

Individuals with Disabilities Education Act (IDEA)

Under IDEA, the federal government provides financial assistance to state and local education agencies in order for these agencies to provide a "free, appropriate public education" to qualifying children with disabilities. In order to be covered by IDEA, a child with diabetes must show that the disease adversely affects his or her educational performance. Once shown, parents and school officials develop an Individualized Education Program (IEP).

In addition to these federal laws, some state laws provide additional protections.

Your Rights

As the parent or legal guardian of a child with diabetes, you have the right

- To have your child assessed under IDEA and/or Section 504.

- To hold an IEP or a Section 504 meeting with school and school district personnel. You have the right to bring an advocate, attorney, and/or experts to this meeting to better explain your child's diabetes management.

- To develop an IEP or a Section 504 plan that specifically states your child's needs and the services required to meet these needs. You do not have to sign the plan if you do not agree with it. To begin implementation, you can sign the parts you agree with and not sign the parts that still require discussion.

- To be notified of any proposed changes in your child's plan, to attend any meetings concerning proposed changes, and to approve any changes.

Addressing Discrimination

Educate

Educate your school personnel about diabetes and how it affects your child. This is often achieved through a combination of the Section 504/IEP process and training selected staff in the specific acts necessary to accommodate your child's needs.

Negotiate

During the process of developing your child's accommodation plan, you may need to negotiate with school officials. You do not have to sign a plan unless you agree to it. However, you are likely to reach agreement more easily if you attempt to understand the concerns of school personnel and negotiate toward an agreement suitable to everyone involved.

Litigate

If your child's needs are not being met, your have the right to file an administrative complaint or a lawsuit in court. The procedure you follow will vary depending on whether your claim is under the IDEA, Section 504, or the Americans with Disabilities Act. After exhausting your other options, seeking protection in the courts may be necessary to ensure that your child receives the education and medical care that he or she deserves.

Legislate

If you find that the current laws and policies aren't providing your child—and other children with diabetes—with the protection they need, your next step might be working to change the rules at either a local, statewide, or national level.

Accommodations

Schools and day care centers covered by the laws discussed in this [section] must accommodate the special needs of qualifying children. Parents should document this accommodation in either a Section 504 plan, an IEP, or as written accommodations under the Americans with Disabilities Act. The document should specifically state the child's disability, needs, accommodations, and how these accommodations will be delivered.

Your written plan might include accommodations such as

- Assuring that there are staff members trained in testing blood glucose levels, recognizing and treating hypoglycemia and hyperglycemia, and administering insulin and glucagon.

- Allowing your child to self-administer blood glucose tests in the classroom and in other locations, and allowing your child to promptly treat hypoglycemia and hyperglycemia.

- Insuring full participation in all sports, extracurricular activities, and field trips, with the necessary assistance and/or supervision provided.

- Eating whenever and wherever necessary, including eating lunch at an appropriate time with enough time to finish eating.

- Taking extra trips to the bathroom or water fountain.

- Permitting extra absences for medical appointments and sick days when necessary.

These are examples of some of the things to include in an individual plan. Consult with your child's health care team when determining your child's requirements.

Schools Database

You easily can find out whether your child's school allows blood testing in the classroom and whether there is a full-time nurse at the school by using the Internet or e-mail. A Web site that maintains a schools database with this information can be accessed at *ChildrenWithDiabetes.com*. The information is available for free using your computer. You also can add information or comments on the school's blood testing policy or availability of the school nurse to the database if you wish.

Access the database at *www.ChildrenWithDiabetes.com/schools/*. If you cannot find your child's school listed, you can send an e-mail to *info@ChildrenWithDiabetes.com* and include the school's name, address and NCES ID, which is the unique four- or five-digit number that is assigned to every U.S. public school. The Web site also offers further information about educating students and school personnel, as well as checklists and forms that you are free to print out and use.

7

Children's Camp

Special Diabetes Camps

Children with diabetes have unique problems that challenge them at each stage of their growth. Summer camps such as the Florida Camp for Children and Youth with Diabetes (FCCYD) provide diabetic children with a camping experience that is fun, supportive and educational.

In the early years, camp personnel teach campers to accurately and routinely check their blood glucose levels and to administer their own insulin injections. The importance of diet and exercise is emphasized. Emotional and psychological adjustment problems reach their peak during the adolescent years. For all of these stages, Florida's Diabetes Camp has developed programming to help the child and family.

Special summer camp has been held every August at various north Florida locations. To the eye of the casual observer, it looks like any other camp.

For about three weeks (divided into two sessions), a couple of hundred kids ranging in age from seven to fourteen years old participate in a wide variety of activities. They swim, sail, canoe across a lake and run in relay races. They do crafts, sit around a campfire singing songs and telling stories, all this while their parents get some well-deserved rest.

Earlier in the summer, over a route nearly 100 miles long through northern Florida, a group of older teenagers (fifteen to twenty) spend the better part of a week cycling, scuba diving and setting up tents at nightfall. This group, like the children at camp, are normal, well-adjusted kids enthusiastically taking part in strenuous activities, burning off the excess energy that results from being out of school.

What they all have in common, though, is something that sets them apart from other children. Every morning they all have to pull out a syringe, alcohol swabs and a bottle of insulin and inject themselves with the prescribed insulin. They all have diabetes.

The FCCYD runs both the summer camp for children and the "adventure camp" for teens. The camp is the only one of its kind in the state.

Camping experiences for children and youth with diabetes are invaluable.

Camp is a place where the children learn self-confidence and independence. Camps provide exciting outdoor activities while teaching the kids to manage their diabetes successfully.

Many camps provide financial assistance to help children who are unable to pay the full camp fee. There are camps all over the United States.

For more information on camps near you, contact your local chapter of the American Diabetes Association, or log onto *http://www.diabetes.org/ada/camps.htm.*

8

Child Care Providers

Finding a provider

Trying to find a child care provider who is competent enough to take care of a child with diabetes can be difficult. To find someone experienced with diabetes, try contacting your local hospital, physician, diabetes nurse educator, or the American Diabetes Association. Other ways to locate the right babysitter are through religious organizations, neighbors or the parents of other diabetic children.

If you live out in the country as we do, it becomes even more difficult to find a sitter. We decided to look for someone mature whom we liked and could trust with our children and home. When we found the right person, we gave her written information and a tape on diabetes. After she looked over all the information, I would quiz her on it. Then we would practice giving injections, pricking fingers and familiarizing her with where all the medications were and what foods she would need. I explained to her about hypoglycemia and hyperglycemia.

After the initial training was over, I would leave her with the children for just a couple of hours at a time. Also, I would put their snacks in a zip-lock plastic bag so I could control the amount of carbohydrates they got.

Educating our child care provider was the best thing we ever did. Now if I need to leave the children with the sitter, I am confident that they are being well taken care of. It may be time consuming to find and educate a sitter, but the rewards are great. All parents deserve time away occasionally to refresh themselves, and it is also good for the children to be with other caring adults.

Instruction sheets

Where I am: _____

My pager number: _____

Husband's pager number: _____

Hospital number: _____

Neighbor's name & number: _____

Doctor's name & number: _____

Time for monitoring blood sugars: _____

Time for injections: _____

What dose of insulin is needed N _____ H_____ R _____

Time for snacks: _____

Time for lunch: _____   Time for dinner: _____

Time for bath: _____

Time for play: _____

Time for bed: _____

What they can and cannot do: _____

_____

_____

_____

_____

_____

Special instructions

• • • Always treat right away if their blood sugar is low • • •

Extremely Low:
(If their blood glucose is 40 or below)
Treat with 1 4-oz. juice or 1 8-oz. Gatorade box drink
            2 glucose tablets
            2 peanut butter crackers

Moderately Low:
(If their blood glucose is 41 to 55)
Treat with 1 4-oz. juice or 1 8-oz. Gatorade box drink
            1 glucose tablets
            2 peanut butter crackers

Low:
(If their blood glucose is 56 to 69)
Treat with 1 4-oz. juice or 1 8-oz. Gatorade box drink
            1 peanut butter cracker

NOTE: May follow up with a blood glucose test 20-30 minutes later if the child is still feeling bad.

When their blood glucose is too low (less than 70), treat them. When their blood glucose is too high (greater than 240), check for ketones and call the parents.

9

Sick Days

DEALING WITH SICK DAYS can be difficult and frustrating. When the child comes down with a cold or the flu, don't be surprised if blood sugar levels are higher and ketones are present in the urine. When children become ill, their bodies usually require more insulin.

The first rule to battling any illness is to continue taking insulin. If the child is vomiting and not eating, insulin is still required. You need to contact the doctor or nurse. Also, a child may have ketones when blood sugar levels are low. So it is important to monitor the blood sugar levels and to check for ketones more frequently in times of illness.

With any illness, it is important to drink plenty of fluids to keep hydrated. If the child is urinating more frequently because blood sugar levels are elevated, even more fluids are required. Remember, staying well hydrated will help avoid the fluid loss that occurs when the child is vomiting or has diarrhea. When the child becomes too dehydrated, intravenous fluid replacement may be required.

Both of our children have had to be admitted to the hospital for intravenous fluid replacement at times. When they had a virus that lasted for 24 hours, we tried to give them fluids by mouth, but they could not keep the fluids down. Vomiting continued for six hours and their sugar levels kept dropping into the low 40s. The nurse had to administer an IV with saline and glucose. By the next day both children were doing well and were able to return home.

Below are a few examples of what you can do to help yourself and your child get through the sick days:

- Check glucose levels every two to four hours.
- Check for ketones (240mg/dl and over) a couple of times a day even when blood sugar levels are low.
- Always give them insulin. Usually I have to change the amount of insulin according to their illness and what the doctor says.
- Give them plenty of fluids.
- Read some good books to them!

Helpful supplies:

- Phenergan suppositories for nausea and vomiting.
- Feverall over-the-counter suppositories to reduce fever and pain.
- Tylenol for fever (temp. less than 101.5 degrees F or 38.5 degrees C).
- Triaminic Syrup for cold and allergies (orange flavor) and Triaminic Expectorant for chest and head congestion (citrus flavor).
- Dimetapp Cold & Allergy relieves nasal congestion, runny nose, itchy, watery eyes and sneezing.
- Emetrol – available without a prescription. Helps settle the stomach (use as directed).
- Pepto Bismol for upset stomachs.
- Thermometer.

- Luden's Sugar-Free Wild Cherry Throat Drops for a sore throat.
- N'ICE Sugar-Free Lozenges relieves sore throats and coughs.
- Nasal decongestant spray helps clear a stuffy nose.

NOTE: *Always check with your physician before you give the child any kind of medication.*

Managing an upset stomach:

- When the child is nauseated or has vomited, feed only ice chips until the nausea clears. When the child feels a little better, small sips of fluids should be taken slowly. (I usually give my children small sips of juice every 5 minutes).

- Flat carbonated Sprite or 7-Up is good to sip on if the child's blood sugar level is low. If it is above 240mg/dl, then you should give them flat diet drinks. You can add a little warm water to the soda to help eliminate the carbonation more quickly.

- Natural apple sauce, Jello or clear soup broth can be given. Some sugar is needed as a fuel source to keep the body from breaking down fat and muscle tissue.

- Common sense should always prevail! Crackers and toast are good choices to feed a child after he or she is feeling better. Introduce their usual diet slowly. Avoid spicy, greasy or fatty foods.

NOTE: *If the vomiting persists for more than a couple of hours, call the doctor.*

10

Exercise

EXERCISE IS CRITICAL to ensure good blood glucose control. A regular exercise program is essential for everyone to maintain a healthy body. People with diabetes should exercise on a daily basis. We need to encourage children to go out and play tag, kickball, run, etc. When they get the exercise they need, you will see a tremendous difference in their blood sugar levels. Our children exercise on a daily schedule.

Daily exercise yields many benefits:
- Helps keep blood sugar levels in the desired range
- Helps body cells become more sensitive to insulin
- Improves muscle tone
- Helps reduce stress level
- Results in more energy and increases the body's metabolic rate
- Helps to reduce appetite
- Causes one to increase fluid intake
- Improves one's concentration

- Helps one sleep better
- Helps one lose or control his/her weight
- Makes one feel better

Walking and jogging

Walking and jogging are safe and effective ways of improving physical fitness. Walking can increase the efficiency of the heart and lungs, help lower blood sugar levels and help decrease blood pressure.

Before children start walking or jogging, it is important to get them a good pair of shoes. Shoes should be lightweight and fit comfortably. They should also provide good arch support, plenty of width in the toe area, a well-cushioned midsole and heel to absorb shock.

Before they start, make sure they do stretching exercises for at least five minutes before walking to gradually increase their heart rates, loosen up the joints and stretch the muscles. After they finish, they should cool down by walking slowly and then stretching for five or more minutes.

Try to make the exercise routine the same time each day. A good time to walk or jog is after breakfast or after dinner. Before they start and finish, make sure you monitor their blood sugar level to be sure that it is not too low.

Exercise for children

Too many children spend much more time playing video games than playing tag. Parents often drive their children to their neighbors' houses instead of letting them walk or ride their bikes. The average child spends 25 hours per week watching TV. One study found that 32 percent of fourth-graders watch six or more hours of television a day. Little daily exercise also contributes to the increasing rates of obesity among school-age children. Inactive lifestyles are not good for the children's health. Parents need to be more aware of how their children spend their time.

These exercises are wonderful for children:

- Running
- Swimming
- Bicycling
- Jumping Rope
- Gymnastics
- Soccer
- Basketball
- Playing Tag
- Golf
- Trampoline
- Kick Ball
- Dodge Ball
- Tennis
- Walking
- Volleyball
- Softball
- Skateboarding
- Roller Blading/Skating

Like adults, most kids do not want to exercise. The great thing about playing sports is that the children do not realize that they are exercising. Getting them outside and playing is the key. Just be sure you know what their blood sugar levels are before they go out and play hard. If the levels are on the low side, then give them a snack. Always send them out with glucose tablets or regular hard candy because their blood sugar levels could drop too low and they might not be able to get back home quickly enough. Always have them take some food supplies along.

It is important for all diabetics, regardless of their age, to listen to their bodies for warning signs such as headache, nausea, stomachache, shakiness or dizziness. When these symptoms occur, you must treat the reaction quickly. Do not wait.

As soon as the children begin to feel poorly, they should stop, eat and rest. Once they feel better, then they can continue to play or exercise.

What works best for our children when we go out and play is for one of us to carry a waist pouch with two 4-oz. box juices, a couple of glucose tablets and one pack of six peanut butter crackers. When the children feel low, they stop right away and drink the juice first and then eat some crackers. A snack should consist of something to raise the blood sugar immediately, followed by a complex carbohydrate (such as a cracker) and protein (such as peanut butter or cheese) to maintain the blood glucose level.

After school, our children do their homework and then they go outside and play. After dinner we go outside as a family and walk, play ball, run or play on the trampoline.

On the weekends, the children go outside and play in the mid-morning and again in the afternoon. If the weather is bad, they stay inside and we play exercise games instead.

Rainy-day activities

On rainy days when you and your family cannot go outside and exercise, do some fun exercise games inside.

Exercise add-on

Have your family stand in a circle. Have one child do an exercise of his or her choice, such as jumping jacks. The next person then performs the jumping jacks and one other exercise. This routine continues around the circle.

Clothespin Hunt

Similar to an Easter egg hunt. Write down some exercise instructions on pieces of paper and clothespins in different places. Make up about fifteen different exercises and put them on the pieces of paper with the clothespins. To find a clothespin you must walk fast, not slowly. Every time someone finds a clothespin, all the family members do the exercise for 30 seconds.

Giant Steps and Hops and Baby Steps and Hops

Choose one person to be the commander and stand at the end of a large area or a long hallway. Tell the children to take one or two giant steps, one or two giant hops, one or two baby steps and one or two baby hops. Whoever reaches the commander first gets to be commander next.

Copy the Leader

Turn on some kids' music. Have the children copy everything the leader does. Do all kinds of exercises. The children will exercise immediately. They love this game.

Follow the Captain

Choose a leader. Everyone stands in a line behind the leader, about three feet apart. The leader stretches as high as he can, kicks legs, wiggles arms, does some somersaults, jumping jacks, jiggles legs, etc. Everyone imitates the leader. Play this for about 15 minutes.

Partner Bicycle Pumps

Both children sit on the floor facing each other. Make sure that their soles and heels are touching each other. Now partners start to bicycle pump, keeping their feet in contact with one another. Go slowly for awhile, then faster for awhile, then even faster. Time how long they can do it.

Running and Jumping

The first person starts running in place for thirty seconds, then gets a jump rope and jumps rope for another thirty seconds. While they are running in place, the other person counts how many times their legs moved and then how many times they jumped rope. Everyone takes a turn. You can increase the time depending on the age of the children.

Leap and Hit

You will need a ball and a hoop or some tape. Place the hoop or tape on the floor and someone on the other side of the hoop holding the ball up high. The other person runs toward you, jumps into the center of the hoop (or a target spot marked on the floor with the tape) and then leaps up to hit the ball from your hands. Make sure you hold the ball within his reach so he does not become frustrated and lose interest. As the child gets more proficient, you can raise the ball's height.

Balloon Volleyball

Get some tape or some string and place it on the floor for your net. Use a balloon for your volleyball. You can hit the balloon three times to help get it over.

Radio/CD Player/Headphones

Encourage adolescents to "dance to the music" to increase their activity level.

Trampoline Jumping

For the older, more coordinated child, a small round indoor trampoline may provide an appealing alternative on a rainy day.

Since the children have become more active, their blood sugar levels are much closer to normal. It does take more time in some ways. We must watch that they are exercising enough and that their blood sugar levels do not drop too low. When they do exercise strenuously, the children usually require a larger snack. Also, encourage the children to drink plenty of water before, during and after playing. It is truly important to instill in them the idea that exercise is a vital part of managing diabetes. Make exercise a game with your family. Enjoy all the wonderful times together because life is so short and precious.

11

Nutrition

EVERYBODY TALKS ABOUT NUTRITION these days. I never really thought about it as much as I do now. Nutrition is important, not just for my children, but for everyone. The fat content of the food we eat is just as important as the amount of sugar we consume.

Carbohydrates are molecules made up of many sugars linked together. When carbohydrates are digested in the body, they eventually are broken down into simple sugars.

The body has several ways of using carbohydrates that have been changed into glucose (blood sugar). Energy can be formed to fuel the body; fuel energy in the liver for emergency use can be formed; and fuel energy in the muscles can be made for future exercise. Any remaining glucose is either stored in fat cells or passed through the urine.

Protein is essential for growth and development. It provides the body with energy, which is needed for growth, antibodies, enzymes, and muscle tissues. Only protein can make new cells to replace worn out or damaged cells. Protein is found in meats, fish, poultry, milk, cheese and eggs. Insufficient protein intake can result in stunted growth, diarrhea, vomiting, lack of appetite and edema (a buildup of fluids in the tissues).

It does not matter whether one has diabetes or not—everyone should eat more whole grains, fruits and vegetables. Everybody should avoid indulging in cakes, candies, ice cream and sugars in excess.

Developing a diet

A diet for a person with diabetes can be developed using several different methods. The most common are exchange lists, carbohydrate counting, or a combination of both.

All diets are developed based on the required number of calories per day. The doctor will provide this information based on your child's age, height and present weight. He or she may also refer you to a registered dietitian (RD), who can explain an appropriate diet to you. Some RDs are also Certified Diabetes Educators (CDE). A CDE has advanced training in diet therapy education for diabetes.

The usual diabetes diet is divided into 50-60 percent carbohydrates (CHO), 20-25 percent protein (P), and 20-25 percent fat (F). The doctor or dietitian will give you the actual percentage of each food type.

Exchange list

The exchange list is the most commonly used for planning a diet. The amount of carbohydrates, protein and fat content will vary.

Below is a chart of the exchange list for starch/bread, meat, vegetable, fruit, milk and fat. These items have been broken down into grams of carbohydrates, proteins, fats and calories. (Grams are weight measurements that are smaller than ounces.)

In addition to understanding the content of food, portion control also must be watched. The amount you eat of a particular food is also important in developing the best diet for your needs.

Exchange List

	Carbohydrate (g)	Protein (g)	Fat (g)	Calories
Starch/Bread	15	3	trace	80
Meat				
Lean	–	7	3	55
Medium-Fat	–	7	5	75
High-Fat	–	7	8	100
Vegetable	15	2	–	25
Fruit	15	–	–	60
Milk				
Skim	12	8	trace	90
Low fat	12	8	5	120
Whole	12	8	8	150

Through the years it has been difficult to keep my children's blood sugar levels stable. They were constantly fluctuating between too high and too low. Day by day I would get so discouraged, until one day I met a wonderful lady named Theo Reed. She has worked for fifteen years at the V.A. Hospital in Lake City, Florida. She is an Advanced Registered Nurse Practitioner (ARNP) and a Certified Diabetes Educator (CDE).

Theo explained to me the importance of counting carbohydrates for children...or anyone with diabetes. I spent many weeks learning how to weigh foods, counting out the children's snacks per serving and reading all the food labels. This was time-consuming in the beginning, but it became easier with time. Now I can look at a potato, for example, and tell you about how many carbohydrates are in it because it is a food item that we eat often.

Our diet has worked out well for us. The children's hemoglobin (A1C) has been outstanding. It has been ranging between 6.0 and 7.1. I believe our diet has helped me keep their blood sugar levels in a good range. It does take a lot more time, but it is well worth it. An added benefit is the improved diet of the other family members—those without diabetes. Healthy eating becomes a way of life for everyone in the family.

Counting carbohydrates

This approach to diet requires that you count only the grams of carbohydrates (the sugar and starch of your food). This method gives you more flexibility than any other. It also allows you the freedom and control to adjust the amount of different kinds of foods and even to include foods that were once forbidden to a person with diabetes.

If you look at the exchange list, you will see that there are carbohydrates in the starch and fruit list. Do you remember that there are carbohydrates in vegetables and milk? You can use the exchange list to start counting carbohydrates. Each food portion in the starch, fruit, vegetable and milk groups contains approximately twelve to fifteen grams of carbohydrates. There is even more flexibility if you use the actual carbohydrate grams given on the food labels and food charts and in many recipes.

Before beginning this type of diet plan, you will need recipes, food charts or food labels that list CHO in grams. You also will need measuring spoons, cups and a scale that is calibrated in ounces. Measure or weigh food portions when you are starting out. At first, it is difficult to judge the size of food servings accurately, but they affect blood sugar control greatly. If the child is on a 1200 calorie diet, for example, the carbohydrates (CHO) should make up 50 percent, protein 25 percent and fat 25 percent. The calories are to be distributed among three meals and three snacks. Use this information to calculate the CHO grams for each meal.

The following is a step-by-step example of how I have used CHO counting:

1. Calculate calories for carbohydrates, protein and fat using a 1200-calorie diet.

    50% carbohydrates
        1,200 calories multiplied by 50% =   600 calories
    25% protein
        1,200 calories multiplied by 25% =   300 calories
    25% fat
        1,200 calories multiplied by 25% =   300 calories
                                         ————————

    TOTAL =   1,200 calories

    (Sometimes the grand total will add up to a few more or fewer calories than prescribed, but this is not a problem.)

2. Using the calories, calculate the total grams of CHO needed daily. CHO makes the greatest difference in blood sugar. No one knows exactly how much protein or fat is changed into blood sugar, but it is a small amount. Also, the change takes several hours; because of this, protein and fat are not factored into CHO counting.

    One gram of CHO = 4 calories
    600 calories divided by 4 = 150 grams of CHO

3. Calculate how many grams of CHO should be in each meal or snack. These amounts will need to be adjusted based on trial and error, observation of the child's response to diet, insulin dose, exercise, different foods and his or her blood sugar test results. As a general rule, make changes slowly (not every day unless there is an urgent need). Patience, time and experience are necessary for this to work. The usual diet for children begins with three meals and three snacks.

150 grams of CHO daily may be allocated like this:

Breakfast 25%   (150 multiplied by 25%) = 37.50 grams
Midmorning Snack 10% (150 multiplied by 10%) = 15.00 grams
Noon Meal 25%   (150 multiplied by 25%) = 37.50 grams
Midafternoon Snack 10% (150 multiplied by 10%) = 15.00 grams
Evening Meal 20%   (150 multiplied by 20%) = 30.00 grams
Bedtime Snack 10%   (150 multiplied by 10%) = 15.00 grams

$$$$ 150.00 grams
(CHO)

4. Use the CHO allotted for each meal. You may use the
    CHO values in the exchange list system, but many times
    you have to estimate either grams or the portions. To get
    the best blood sugar control, use food charts and espe-
    cially the food labels.

Sample Menus

Sample Menu 1
Breakfast
Cheerios	¾ cup	=	18 grams
Bread (wheat light)	1 slice	=	9 grams
Milk (1% low fat)	¾ to 1 cup	=	10 grams
			37 grams

Midmorning Snack
Cheez–it (reduced fat)	25 pcs.	=	15 grams
Water	1 cup	=	0 grams
			15 grams

Lunch

Bread (wheat light)	2 slices	=	18 grams
Turkey (deli)	3 slices	=	0 grams
Swiss cheese	1 slice	=	0 grams
Grapes	¾ cup	=	12 grams
Pretzels	9 pcs.	=	7 grams
water		=	0 grams
			37 grams

Midafternoon Snack

Apple	1 medium	=	14 grams
Cottage cheese	¼ cup	=	2 grams
water		=	0 grams
			16grams

Dinner

Baked chicken breast	1 piece	=	0 grams
Carrots (steamed)	½ cup	=	8 grams
Potato	1 med	=	15 grams
Bun	1	=	7 grams
Sugar-free punch	1 cup	=	0 grams
			30 grams

Bedtime Snack

Vanilla wafer cookie	2	=	5 grams
Banana	1 med	=	10 grams
Water	1 cup	=	0 grams
			15 grams

Total carbohydrates	=	150 grams

Sample Menu 2

Breakfast

Corn tortilla	1	=	15 grams
Mexican cheese	2 oz.	=	0 grams
Apple juice	4 oz.	=	15 grams
			33 grams

Midmorning Snack

Mango, small	1 fruit	=	15 grams
Water	1 cup	=	0 grams
			15 grams

Lunch

Pozole (pork and hominy soup)	1 cup	=	22 grams
with shredded cabbage	½ cup	=	3 grams
Lime juice	1 tbsp.	=	1 gram
Flour tortilla	1	=	15 grams
Water, diet soda or iced tea	8 oz.	=	0 grams
			41 grams

Midafternoon Snack

Orange, small	1	=	15 grams
Peanuts	1 oz.	=	0 grams
water		=	0 grams
			15 grams

Dinner

Boiled beans	⅓ cup	=	15 grams
Mexican rice	⅓ cup	=	15 grams
Chicken	4 oz.	=	0 grams
with mole sauce	½ cup	=	5 grams
Water, diet soda or iced tea	8 oz.	=	0 grams
			35 grams

Bedtime Snack

Milk, non-fat	4 oz.	=	6 grams
Banana	½	=	8 grams
			14 grams

Total carbohydrates	=	150 grams

Sample Menu 3

Breakfast

Grits	½ cup	=	15 grams
Biscuit	1	=	15 grams
Egg	1	=	0 grams
Margarine	1 tsp.	=	0 grams
Milk, non-fat	4 oz.	=	6 grams
			36 grams

Midmorning Snack

Orange, small	1	=	15 grams

Lunch

Green beans	½ cup	=	5 grams
Baked ham	2 oz.	=	0 grams
Mashed potatoes	1 cup	=	30 grams
Lettuce and tomato	1 cup	=	5 grams
Italian salad dressing	1 tbsp.	=	0 grams
Water, diet soda or lemonade	8 oz.	=	0 grams
			40 grams

Midafternoon Snack

Fruit cup (light syrup or no sugar)	½ cup	=	15 grams

Dinner

Baked fish	4 oz.	=	0 grams
Collard greens (seasoned with broth)	½ cup	=	5 grams
Cornbread	2-inch cube	=	15 grams
Sweet potato	½ cup	=	15 grams
Water, diet soda or diet lemonade	8 oz.	=	0 grams
			35 grams

Bedtime Snack

Buttermilk	1 cup	=	12 grams
Total carbohydrates		=	153 grams

Reading the food label

The label lists the nutritional value of foods in grams. The grams of carbohydrates are essential for people with diabetes to control their diet and blood sugar. The numbers in the daily value percentage column are based on a 2000-calorie diet. If your children are supposed to consume a different number of calories per day, then those values will not apply to their diets. Also, the daily value percentage values *do not* add up to 100 percent.

Nutrition Facts

Serving Size 1 1/2 cups (30g)
Servings Per Container about 5

Amount Per Serving

Calories	130
Calories from Fat	30

	% Daily Value*
Total Fat 3.5g	5%
Saturated Fat 0.5g	3%
Cholesterol 0mg	0%
Sodium 380mg	16%
Total Carbohydrate 23g	8%
Sugars 2g	
Protein 2g	

Not a significant source of dietary fiber, vitamin A, vitamin C, calcium and iron.

*Percent Daily Values are based on a 2,000 calorie diet. Your daily values may be higher or lower depending on your calorie needs:

		Calories:	2,000	2,500
Total Fat	Less than		65g	80g
Sat Fat	Less than		20g	25g
Cholesterol	Less than		300mg	300mg
Sodium	Less than		2,400mg	2,400mg
Total Carbohydrate			300g	375g
Dietary Fiber			25g	30g

Calories per gram: Fat 9 • Carbohydrate 4 • Protein 4

Fat

The body does need fats but only the right fats, and only in the correct amounts. The current recommendation is for 30 percent of total calories to come from fat. The exception is for infants, who require a lot more fat in their diets in order to develop properly.

Your body requires fatty acids to carry fat-soluble vitamins, which are essential for growth and development and for maintenance of healthy skin, hair, and nails. Fatty acids also provide the body with energy. A variety of problems occur when the body fails to receive the correct amount of fatty acids. Signs of a fatty acid deficiency may include retarded growth or skin, hair, and nail disorders.

Fat is necessary. Most of us are aware that there are different kinds of dietary fat: saturated, polyunsaturated, and monounsaturated. It is best to limit the amount of fat you eat. Choose mostly monounsaturated fats, because they increase your level of HDL and lower total blood cholesterol. There is no need for large amounts of saturated fat in your diet.

If you use fat substitutes, you can significantly reduce the family's fat intake. Oils from animal products and some plant products (such as coconut, palm and kernel oil) are solid, rather than liquid at room temperature. Examples include meat fat, cream, butter, cheese, whole milk, pork, poultry skin, and shortening. These saturated fats increase your risk of heart disease and also raise the "bad" LDL blood cholesterol more then anything else in your diet.

Oils from vegetable products are liquid at room temperature. Examples include sunflower, corn, safflower and soybean oils. These polyunsaturated fats, in moderation, tend to lower both HDL and LDL blood cholesterol and are helpful in removing cholesterol from the body. Substituting these fats in moderation, instead of saturated fats in your diet, can reduce your risk of heart disease.

Cholesterol is a white, waxy, fatty substance found in all foods that come from animals. Cholesterol is essential to our well-being because it helps build cell membranes, produces hormones, and is essential in the manufacture of bile acids.

The liver is capable of manufacturing most of the cholesterol the body needs. The cholesterol manufactured by the liver is carried through the bloodstream by low-density lipoproteins (LDLs). High levels of LDLs in the bloodstream can result in clogged arteries, causing high blood pressure, stroke or heart disease. This is why LDL is referred to as the "bad" cholesterol.

High-density lipoproteins (HDLs) carry excess cholesterol from different body tissues to the liver, where it is converted to bile acids and then eliminated through the intestines. High levels of HDLs are linked with a decreased risk of coronary heart disease. That is why HDL often is called the "good" cholesterol.

It is important to watch your fat intake because people with diabetes have a high risk of heart disease and strokes. We use this formula below to calculate the fat calories per gram:

Nutrition Information Per Serving: (from food label)

*Grams of fat per serving: _____
*Total calories per serving:_____

Read the nutritional label and look for the number of grams of fats in one serving. Multiply the grams of fat by 9 and then divide by the number of calories per serving. Next, multiply by 100. This exercise will help you determine the percentage of fat in one serving.

Example: Grams of fat x 9
             Calories in one serving

Making a "fat" difference in your diet

Researchers have documented the fact that more than anything else you eat, excess saturated fat can raise the level of cholesterol in the blood. This fact is particularly important because a high level of cholesterol in the blood increases the risk of developing heart disease—the leading cause of death in the United States.

We are careful about how much fat we eat each day. A person with diabetes already has a higher risk of heart disease and stroke. So I feel that we should educate our children on how they can keep their fat intake to a minimum. Below is an outline of ways to help you select foods that are lower in fat.

1. **Read the food labels.**

2. **Limit intake of added fats.**
   Butter, margarine, salad dressings and cooking oils have about fifteen grams of fat per tablespoon. Use a low-fat or a non-fat substitute instead. There are many reduced-fat products on the market now.

*1 gram of fat contains 9 calories

3. **Eat lean meats.**

   Substitute lower-fat cuts of meat for those high in fat.

4. **Eat poultry instead of red meat.**

   Chicken and turkey usually have less fat than beef or pork. Poultry-based luncheon meats and ground meat contain less than 15 percent fat.

5. **Trim and skin poultry and meat.**

   Remove all visible fat from meat and poultry before cooking. Also, remove the skin from poultry.

6. **Limit portions of meat.**

   Limit your intake of meat and poultry to less than 3 ounces per serving or 6 ounces per day.

7. **Eat more fish.**

   Fish is lower in fat, especially saturated fat, than red meat and poultry. Eat fish a couple of times a week.

8. **Eat water-packed tuna.**

   Tuna packed in water has significantly less fat and fewer calories than oil-packed tuna.

9. **Eat low-fat dairy products.**

   Be selective when choosing dairy products. Use skim milk or 1-percent milk, for example, instead of whole or 2-percent milk. Use no-fat or low-fat yogurt instead of whole-milk yogurt or sour cream. If you eat cheese, choose a type that has fewer than 6 grams of fat per ounce.

10. **Eat vegetable protein foods.**

    Dry beans and peas are low in fat and high in both protein and soluble fiber.

11. **Limit your intake of nuts and seeds.**

Although nuts and seeds have protein and fiber, both
are high in fat.

12. **Eat complex carbohydrates.**

Replace foods high in fat with no- or low-fat starchy food
such as pasta, whole-grain breads, rice, vegetables, and cereals.

13. **Eat fruits and vegetables.**

Eat at least five or six servings a day of fruit and vegetables.
Both are high in essential vitamins, minerals and fiber.

14. **Eat low-fat breads.**

Some breads, such as croissants, are high in fat—usually saturated fat. Read the label and try to select low-fat breads such
as bagels.

15. **Limit your intake of fried foods.**

Eat foods that have been baked, broiled, grilled, steamed, mi-
crowaved or roasted instead of fried. If you must eat fried foods,
try patting them with a paper towel to remove excess grease.

16. **Use vegetable coating sprays.**

Coat your non-stick skillet with a vegetable spray instead of
oil, butter, or margarine.

17. **Use unsaturated fats for cooking.**

Unsaturated fats (monounsaturated and polyunsaturated) are
found primarily in vegetable oils (such as peanut, olive,
canola, sunflower, and corn oils). Unsaturated fats have been
found to reduce cholesterol levels in some
individuals.

18. **Limit intake of chocolate.**

Substitute cocoa, which has less fat, for chocolate.

Fat content of foods

It is truly amazing to see how much fat we consume in a day. Most of us do not realize the amount of fat in each food product we eat. Here is a list of the fat percentages of various foods:

100% FAT
Bacon fat, butter, corn oil, lard, margarine, mayonnaise, peanut oil, shortening, soybean oil, wheat germ oil.

90-100% FAT
Artichoke hearts (canned and marinated), bacon, bleu cheese dressing, Brazil nuts, Caesar dressing, cream cheese, Italian dressing, macadamia nuts, olives, pecans, thousand island dressing, whipped cream.

80-90% FAT
Almonds, avocado, bologna, French dressing, fresh coconut, peanut butter, sesame seeds, sour cream, walnuts.

70-80% FAT
Cashews, cheddar cheese, Colby, half-and-half (cream), Monterey Jack, meunster, peanuts, processed American cheese, processed Swiss cheese, pumpkin seeds, some hot dogs, spare ribs, sunflower seeds.

60-70% FAT
American cheese spread, chicken thigh, chuck roast, cream of mushroom soup, cube steak, dried coconut, eggs, liverwurst, mozzarella, pork chop, potato chips, ricotta, salami, Swiss cheese, veal breast.

50-60% FAT
Brownies, chocolate chip cookies, corned beef hash, cream of celery soup, cured shank ham, glazed plain doughnut, ground beef, liver, milk chocolate bar, New England clam chowder, Parmesan cheese, part-skim mozzarella cheese, part-skim ricotta cheese,

porterhouse steak, pound cake, rainbow trout, round steak, salmon, semi-sweet chocolate, T-bone steak.

40–50% FAT
Biscuit, chicken breast, chocolate cake (no icing), cream of potato soup, cured butt ham, custard, danish, French fries, hash browns, ice cream, lamb chops, macaroon, pecan pie, plain cake doughnut, pumpkin pie, sirloin, whole–milk yogurt, whole milk.

30–40% FAT
Apple pie, bran muffins, cheese pizza, chocolate milk, cornbread, creamed cottage cheese, dill pickles, flank steak, fresh ham, granola, lemon meringue pie, low-fat milk, oil-packed tuna, plain waffle, pork and bean soup, tapioca, turkey (dark meat), turkey noodle soup, white cake (no icing), whole-wheat pancakes.

20–30% FAT
Boston cream pie, buttermilk, chocolate pudding, cream of asparagus soup, graham cracker, low-fat yogurt, minestrone, oatmeal-raisin cookie, soda cracker, swordfish, tomato soup, wheat germ.

10–20% FAT
Alfalfa sprouts, broccoli, corn, cottage cheese (2-percent), crab, dinner roll, egg noodles, garbanzo beans, lobster, oatmeal, peanut brittle, plain popcorn, raw wheat bran, red snapper, sherbet, sole, split pea soup, turkey (white meat), whole wheat bread.

0–10% FAT
Apple, apricot, asparagus, baked potato, banana, beets, black beans, brown rice, cantaloupe, carrots, cauliflower, celery, cola, cracked wheat bread, dates, French bread, fruit cocktail, grapefruit, green beans, haddock, halibut, iceberg lettuce, kale, lemon, orange, papaya, peach, pear, peas, pinto beans, plain rice, pretzel, puffed wheat, pumpernickel, red kidney beans, rye, shrimp, skim milk, summer squash, sweet potato, tomato, water-packed tuna, wheat flakes, whole–wheat pasta, yams, yellow corn tortilla.

Our family eats healthier foods now. I think we are better off because we do. We eat less red meat and more fruits and vegetables, and we drink plenty of water. Soda, whether diet, caffeine-free, or regular, is not nutritious for our bodies.

Let us all take care of our bodies today so there will be a tomorrow.

Healthy substitutes

INSTEAD OF:	TRY:
Butter in vegetables	Vegetables with lemon, lime or spices
Sour cream on a baked potato	Cottage cheese, low-fat yogurt or fat-free cheese
Fried Foods	Baked, broiled, steamed, roasted or microwaved
Bacon	Canadian bacon or turkey bacon
Fast-food cheeseburger	Salad or potato bar
Oils, salad dressings, sour cream, mayonnaise	Reduced-calorie salad dressings and sour cream, low-fat or non-fat plain yogurt, mustard
Supermarket baked goodies	Home-baked cookies and cakes using polyunsaturated oils and a lot less sugar
Chips, snack crackers	Crisp breads, pretzels, rice cakes, melba toast, air-popped or microwaved popcorn
Butter	Soft margarine, all-natural jelly

Healthy substitutes

INSTEAD OF:	TRY:
Non-dairy coffee creamer	Skim milk or 1% milk
Cake, pie, cookies, pastries	Fresh fruits, canned fruits in natural juices, baked apples, ginger snaps, graham crackers
Chocolate	Cocoa
Cooking foods with saturated fats	Vegetable oils such as sunflower, olive or peanut oils
Sugar	With most recipes, cutting the sugar by ⅓ cup does not affect the taste. You can eliminate sugar when using apple sauce.
Whole milk	Skim milk, 1% milk, non-fat dry milk or soy milk

Free foods

Free foods have few or no calories and may be used in your meal plan as often as you like. These foods can add color, interest, and texture to your meals and temporarily satisfy hunger.

Beverages
    Club soda
    Crystal Light
    Decaffeinated coffee
    Decaffeinated tea
    Sparkling water, water
    Sugar-free mixed drinks
    Sugar-free soda

Candy
Sugar-free Gummy Bears, taffy, hard candy

Condiments
Kitchen Bouquet*
Mustard*
Pickles, unsweetened*
Spices and herbs
Tabasco sauce
Vinegar

Dessert
Sugar-free gelatin
Sugar-free pudding

Extracts, Flavorings
Almond, vanilla, etc.

Fruits
Cranberries, unsweetened, ½ cup
Rhubarb, unsweetened, ½ cup

Gum
Sugar-free

Spices
If on a sodium-restricted diet, avoid spices containing salt or sodium.

Soup
Bouillon or broth without fat*

Sugar Substitutes
Saccharin (Sweet 'n Low), aspartame (Equal, NutraSweet), sucralose (Splenda)

* High in sodium

Syrup
Sugar-free (1-2 tbsp.)

Vegetables (Raw – 1 cup)
Cabbage
Carrots
Celery
Cucumbers
Green Onions
Mushrooms
Onions
Radishes
Scallions
Zucchini

Foods for moderate use

These foods all have 20 calories or fewer per serving. Because they do contain more calories than "free foods," they need to be limited to three to four choices per day.

Bamboo shoots ($\frac{1}{4}$ cup)
Bean sprouts ($\frac{1}{3}$ cup)
Catsup (1 tbsp.)*
Chili peppers (2 tbsp.)*
Chili sauce (1 tbsp.)*
Cocktail sauce (1 tbsp.)*
Cocoa, dry unsweetened
    powder (1 tbsp.)
Cooking wine ($\frac{1}{4}$ cup)*
Enchilada sauce (2 tbsp.)*
Meat marinade mix ($\frac{1}{8}$ pkg.)*
Pimento (2 tbsp.)*
Red pepper sauce (1 tbsp.)

Salad dressing
   low-calorie (1 tbsp.)
Soy sauce (1 tbsp.)*
Steak sauce (1 tbsp.)*
Stir-fry sauce (1 tbsp.)
Taco sauce (1 tbsp.)*
Teriyaki sauce (1 tbsp.)*
Whipped topping (1 tbsp.)
Worcestershire sauce (1 tbsp.)*
Miller's bran (2 tbsp.)
Non-fat dry milk powder (3 tsp.)

*High in sodium

Foods to watch out for

The following foods can be used in limited amounts. Read the labels for the amount of carbohydrates in each.

Brown sugar
Cakes
Candied fruit
Canned or frozen fruits in heavy syrup
Corn syrup
Doughnuts
Fruit-flavored yogurt
Honey
Jams, preserves
Jelly
Juices sweetened with high fructose syrup
Marshmallows
Molasses
Pies
Powdered sugar
Regular candy (most candy bars)
Regular chewing gum

Regular Jell-O
Regular pudding
Regular soft drinks
Sugar
Sugar-coated cereals
Sweetened condensed milk
Yams in syrup

NOTE: You can use sugar, honey, molasses, etc. if the child has hypo-glycemia (low blood sugar) to help raise the blood sugar level.

Names of sugars

"Beware of these names"

Beet sugar
Brown sugar
Corn Syrup
Dextrose
Fructose
Glucose
Honey
Lactose
Levulose
Malt
Maple sugar
Molasses
Sucrose
Turbinado
Xylose

NOTE: Even though sucralose (which is sold as Splenda) ends in "ose," it has no calories and can be used safely by diabetics. It is made from sugar, but it is not recognized as sugar or carbohydrate by the body.

Food Analysis Charts

FRESH FRUITS

Fruits	Serv. Size	Carbo. (grams)	Protein (grams)	Fat (grams)	Calorie	Vit. C %	Fiber (grams)	Vit. A %
Apple	1 small	18	0	1	80	6	5	★
Banana	1 med.	24	1	1	120	15	3	★
Canteloupe	1 med.	11	1	0	50	90	0	516
Grape	1½ cups	24	1	0	85	9	2	3
Grapefruit	½ med.	14	1	0	50	90	6	32
Honeydew	½ med.	12	1	0	50	40	1	★
Kiwi	2 med.	18	1	1	90	230	4	2
Lemon	1 med.	4	0	0	18	35	0	★
Lime	1 med.	7	0	0	20	35	3	★
Nectarine	1 med.	16	1	1	70	10	3	20
Orange	1 small	13	1	0	50	120	6	★
Papaya	1 med.	30	2	0	117	118	3	612
Peach	2 med.	19	1	0	70	20	1	20
Pear	1 med.	25	1	1	100	10	4	★
Pineapple	2 sl 3" dia	21	1	1	90	35	2	★
Plum	2 med.	17	1	1	70	20	1	9
Strawberry	8 med.	13	1	0	50	140	3	★
Tangerine	2 med.	19	1	0	70	85	2	30
Watermelon	2 cups diced	19	1	0	80	25	1	8

Carbo. = Carbohydrates
★ *less than 1%*

FRESH VEGETABLES

Vegetables	Serv. Size	Carbo. (grams)	Protein (grams)	Fat (grams)	Calorie	Vit. C %	Fiber (grams)	Vit. A %
Asparagus	3.5 ozs.	2	2	0	18	10	2	10
Bell pepper	1 med.	5	1	1	25	130	2	2
Broccoli	5.5 ozs.	4	5	1	40	240	5	10
Cabbage, green	3 ozs.	3	1	0	18	70	2	★
Carrot	1 med.	8	1	1	40	8	1	330
Cauliflower	3 ozs.	3	2	0	18	110	2	★
Celery	4 ozs.	4	1	0	20	15	2	★
Corn, sweet	1 med. ear	17	3	1	75	10	1	5
Cucumber	⅓ med.	3	1	0	18	6	0	4
Green bean	¾ cups	2	1	0	14	8	3	2
Jicama, raw	1 cup	12	1	0	49	★	6	★
Kale greens	½ cup	4	1	0	21	27	★	481
Lettuce, iceberg	3 ozs.	4	1	0	20	4	1	2
Lettuce, leaf	3 ozs.	1	1	0	12	4	1	20
Mushroom	5 med.	3	3	0	25	2	0	★
Nopales, raw (cactus)	1 cup	3	1	0	14	★	2	★
Onion	1 med.	14	1	0	60	20	3	★
Potato	1 med.	23	3	0	110	50	3	★
Squash, summer	½ med.	3	1	0	20	25	1	4
Sweet potato	1 med.	32	2	0	140	50	3	520
Tomato	1 med.	6	1	1	35	40	1	20

Carbo. = Carbohydrates
★ *less than 1%*

FROZEN WAFFLES

Frozen Waffles	Serving Size	Carbo. (grams)	Sugar (grams)
Downy Flake – Buttermilk	2	8	1
Kellogg's Eggo – Buttermilk	2	30	3
Kellogg's Eggo – Common Sense Oat Bran	2	27	3
Kellogg's Eggo – Blueberry	2	33	7
Kellogg's Eggo – Apple Cinnamon	2	33	7
Kellogg's Eggo – Nut & Honey	2	32	7
Kellogg's Eggo Minis – Blueberry	3 sets of 4	32	4
Kellogg's Eggo – Minis	3 sets of 4	34	4
Kellogg's Nutri-Grain Multi Bran	2	32	4
Kellogg's Eggo – Special K	2	29	5

Carbo. = Carbohydrates

HOT CEREAL

Hot Cereal	Serving Size	Carbo. (grams)	Sugar (grams)
Jim Dandy – Quick Grits 5 Minutes	½ cup	35	0
Nabisco – Cream of Rice	¼ cup	38	0
Nabisco – Cream of Wheat, Quick	1 cup	25	0
Quaker Instant Grits – Original	½ cup	22	0
Quaker Instant Grits – Butter	½ cup	21	0
Quaker Instant Grits – Cheddar Cheese	½ cup	21	1
Quaker Instant Grits – Red Eye Gravy & Country	½ cup	21	0
Quaker Multi-Grain Oatmeal	½ cup	29	1
Quaker Oat	½ cup	27	1
Quaker Oat Bran	½ cup	25	1
Sun Country – Quick Oats	½ cup	21	1

Carbo. = Carbohydrates

DRY CEREAL

Dry Cereal	Serving Size	Carbo. (grams)	Sugar (grams)
All Bran – Extra Fiber	½ cup	22	0
All Bran – Original	½ cup	22	5
Cheerios	1 cup	22	1
Clusters	½ cup	20	7
Common Sense – Oat Bran-Kellogg's	¾ cup	23	6
Corn Chex	1¼ cup	26	3
Corn Pops	1 cup	26	3
Crispix (Kellogg's)	1 cup	26	4
Fiber One	½ cup	24	0
Grape Nuts	½ cup	47	7
Grape Nuts – Wheat & Barley	½ cup	47	7
Honey Bunches of Oats w/ Almonds	¾ cup	24	6
Kellogg's Complete Brand Flakes	¾ cup	25	6
Kellogg's Corn Flakes	1 cup	26	2
Kellogg's Rice Krispies	1¼ cup	26	3
Kix (General Mills)	1⅓ cup	26	3
Life (Quaker Oats)	¾ cup	25	6
Multigrain Cheerios	1 cup	23	6
Nabisco 100% Bran	⅓ cup	23	7
Nabisco Shredded Wheat	1 cup	41	0

Dry Cereal *(cont.)*

Dry Cereal	Serving Size	Carbo. *(grams)*	Sugar *(grams)*
Nabisco Shredded Wheat & Bran	1¼ cup	47	1
Nutri-Grain (General Mills)	1 cup	24	2
Nutri-Grain (Golden Wheat)	¾ cup	24	6
Post Bran Flakes	¾ cup	24	6
Product 19	1 cup	25	3
Puffed Kashi	1 cup	19	0
Quaker Toasted Oatmeal Original	¾ cup	25	7
Quaker Oatmeal Squares	1 cup	43	9
Quaker Puffed Rice	1 cup	12	0
Quaker Puffed Wheat	1¼ cup	11	0
Rice Chex	1 cup	27	2
Special K	1 cup	21	3
Total (Whole Grain)	¾ cup	24	5
Total Corn Flakes	1¾ cup	25	3
Wheat Chex	¾ cup	41	5
Wheaties (General Mills)	1 cup	24	4

Carbo. = Carbohydrates

SNACKS

Snacks	Serving Size	Carbo. (grams)	Protein (grams)	Fat (grams)	Sugar (grams)	Calorie
Pepperidge Farm Goldfish Cheddar	1 oz. or 51 pcs.	18	3	5	0	130
Pepperidge Farm Goldfish Original	1 oz. or 51 pcs.	17	3	6	0	130
Pepperidge Farm Goldfish Pretzel	1 oz. or 51 pcs.	20	3	2.5	1	110
Nabisco Snack Well's Snack Crackers						
Zesty Cheese	32 crackers	23	3	2	2	120
Nabisco Cheese Tid-Bit Baked						
Snack Crackers	32 crackers	17	2	8	1	150
Keebler Wheatable Wheat Snack						
Crackers White Cheddar						
Cheese Flavor	25 crackers	18	3	7	2	150
Sunshine Cheez-it Snack						
Crackers	27 crackers	16	4	8	1	160
Nabisco Swiss Cheese Baked						
Snack Crackers	15 crackers	18	2	7	2	140
Nabisco Triscuit Baked						
Whole Wheat Waffers	7 wafers	21	3	5	0	140
Sunshine Krispy Soup						
& Oyster	17 crackers	11	2	1.5	1	60
Sunshine Cheez-it						
Reduced Fat	0 crackers	19	4	4.5	1	140
Betty Crocker Bugles Corn Snack						
Nacho Cheese	1 ⅓ cups	18	2	9	2	160

Carbo. = Carbohydrates

SNACKS *(cont.)*

Snacks	Serving Size	Carbo. (grams)	Protein (grams)	Fat (grams)	Sugar (grams)	Calorie
Nabisco Ritz-Bits Sandwich Real Cheese Snack Crackers	14 sandwiches	17	3	10	4	160
Nabisco Ritz-Bits Sandwich Real Peanut Butter Snack Crackers	14 sandwiches	18	4	8	4	160
Nabisco Graham Crackers	2 whole sheets	22	2	3	7	120
Frito Lay Baked Tostitos	1 oz. or 13 pcs.	24	3	1	0	110
Louise's Fat-Free Potato Chips Original	1 oz. or 30 pcs.	23	3	0	0	110
Nabisco Ritz Air Crisps (Sour Cream & Onion)	24 crackers	22	2	5	3	140
Pepperidge Farm Cinnamon Raisin Crunchy Baked	⅙ of pkg.	19	2	5	1	130
Keebler Munch'ems Chili Cheese	28 crackers	23	3	4	3	140
Nabisco Reduced Fat Wheat Thins	18 crackers	21	2	4	3	120
Nabisco Mr. Phipps Tater Crisps Bar-B-Que	1 oz. or 21 pcs.	21	2	4	3	130
Planters Cheez Curls (Reduced Fat)	1 cup	19	3	5	**	130
Nabisco Ritz Snack Mix Cheddar Cheese	½ cup	21	3	7	2	150
Nabisco Mr. Phipps Tater Crisps Original	23 crisps	20	2	4.5	2	120

Carbo. = Carbohydrates
*** = less than 1 gram*

SNACKS *(cont.)*

Snacks	Serving Size	Carbo. (grams)	Protein (grams)	Fat (grams)	Sugar (grams)	Calorie
Nabisco Ritz Snack Mix						
Traditional Flavor	½ cup	21	2	7	2	150
Nabisco Ritz Ark Animal Crackers	46 crackers	21	2	5	3	140
Keebler Wheatable Wheat Snack						
(50% Reduced Fat)	29 crackers	21	3	3.5	3	130
Nabisco Cheez Nips (Reduced Fat)	31 crackers	21	3	3.5	0	130
Keebler Town House Crackers						
(50% Reduced Fat)	6 crackers	11	1	2	2	70
Nabisco Vegetable Thins	14 crackers	19	2	9	2	160
Nabisco Premium Saltine						
Crackers (Fat-Free)	5 crackers	11	1	0	0	50
Lance Captain's Wafer Crackers	4 crackers	9	1	2.5	1	70
Keebler Honey Graham						
Crackers (Low Fat)	9 crackers	25	2	1.5	9	120
Eagle Pretzel Rods (Fat-Free)	3 pretzels	26	3	0	★★	110
Rold Gold Pretzels (Fat-Free)	18 pretzels	23	3	0	★★	100
Bachman Pretzel Sticks						
(6 1–oz. packs)	1 pack	20	2	1	1	100

Carbo. = Carbohydrates
★★ = less than 1 gram

ICE CREAM, YOGURT AND POPSICLES

Ice Cream, Yogurt, and Popsicles	Serving Size	Carbo. (grams)	Protein (grams)	Fat (grams)	Sugar (grams)	Alcohol Sugar**	Cal.
Nabisco Comet Ice Cream Cones	1 cone	4	0	0	0	0	20
Edy's Marble Fudge (No Sugar Added)	½ cup	15	4	3	3	5	100
Dannon – Light Frozen Yogurt Chocolate	½ cup	21	0	4	5	0	80
Dannon – Light Frozen Yogurt Vanilla	½ cup	21	0	4	6	0	80
Dannon – Light Frozen Yogurt Cherry Vanilla Swirl	½ cup	21	0	3	5	0	90
Dannon – Light Frozen Yogurt Peach Raspberry Melba	½ cup	21	0	4	6	0	90
Bryer's Vanilla (No Sugar Added)	½ cup	12	5	3	4	0	90
Bryer's Vanilla Fudge Twirl (No Sugar Added)	½ cup	16	4	3	4	0	100
Bryer's Vanilla Chocolate Strawberry (No Sugar Added)	½ cup	13	5	3	4	0	100
Edy's Strawberry (No Sugar Added)	½ cup	13	4	3	4	3	90
Edy's Mocha Fudge (No Sugar Added)	½ cup	15	0	3	3	5	100
Nestle Crunch Reduced Fat (No Sugar Added)	1 bar	14	7	3	6	1	130
Weight Watchers Orange Vanilla Treat	2 bars	17	1	4	4	0	70
Dole Fruit Juice Bars (No Sugar Added)	1 bar	6	0	0	3	2	54
Good Humor Sugar-Free Popsicles	1 bar	3	0	0	0	0	15
Eskimo Pie	1 pie	25	7	4	4	0	180
Shurfine Ice Cream Cones	1 cone	20	0	0	0	0	20

Carbo. = Carbohydrates; Cal. = Calorie
** = *Alcohol Sugar: Is part of the artificial sweetener*

COOKIES

Cookies	Serving Size	Carbo. (grams)	Protein (grams)	Fat (grams)	Sugar (grams)	Calorie
Pepperidge Farm Butterscotch						
Oatmeal	per 3 cookies	22	2	9	1	170
Murray Butter	per 8 cookies	20	2	4	5	130
English Toffee	per 2 cookies	16	2	8	4	145
Nabisco Pecan Passion	per 1 cookie	9	1	5	3	90
Golden Bowl Fortune	per 2 cookies	12	1	0	5	56
Frookie Oatmeal Raisin All Natural	per 2 cookies	14	2	0	10	90
Health Valley Fruit Centers						
Raspberry Fat-Free	per 1 cookie	18	2	0	9	70
McKee Foods Little Debbie Animal	1 wrap pack	33	3	5	8	180
Keebler Pecan Sandies Reduced Fat	per 1 cookie	10	1	3	3	70
Keebler Vanilla Wafers Reduced Fat	per 8 cookies	25	2	3.5	11	130
Cookie Lover's Dutch						
Chocolate Chip	per 1 cookie	12	1	4	4	90
Land O Lakes Frosted Butter	per 2 cookies	15	2	8	3	140
Musselman's Apple Sauce Oatmeal	per 3 cookies	25	2	4	9	140
Health English Toffee	per 3 cookies	19	2	10	5	170
Staugger Honey Graham Animal	per 16 cookies	24	2	2	7	120
Nestle Butterfinger	per 3 cookies	18	2	6	8	130

Carbo. = Carbohydrates

Vitamins and supplements

My children take three different types of vitamin supplements each day, including chromium picolinate and high-potency proteolytic enzymes. I truly believe that chromium picolinate has helped reduce their blood glucose levels. I put them on this mineral for one month and during that time, their insulin was reduced by two units. Then they stopped taking chromium and within four to five days, I had to increase their insulin.

Research has found that the nutritional supplement chromium picolinate may aid in controlling diabetes. It is made up of *chromium*, which helps increase the efficiency of insulin, and *picolinate*, an amino acid that allows the body to use chromium more readily.

My children take high-potency proteolytic enzymes after every meal to help digest and break down foods, enabling the nutrients to be absorbed into the bloodstream for use in various bodily functions. They always take their vitamins with food and wash them down with a full glass of water to enhance absorption and ensure that the the nutrients are carried to the cells.

Diabetic patients who take daily chromium picolinate supplements may experience a decline in blood glucose levels. It also may offer an added benefit for overweight diabetic patients because improving the action of insulin helps the body to burn fat more efficiently.

Enzymes are energized protein molecules necessary in virtually all biochemical activities, such as digesting food, stimulating the brain and repairing tissue, including organs and cells. Each enzyme is specific in its body function; no other enzyme can take its place. One enzyme can convert dietary phosphorus into bone, for example, while other enzymes prompt the oxidation of glucose, creating energy for cells. Some important enzymes remove dangerous waste materials from the bloodstream by converting them into easily-eliminated substances.

Enzymes are divided into two groups: *digestive* and *metabolic*. Digestive enzymes can be broken down further into three main categories: *amylase*, *protease* and *lipase*. Amylase, which is found in saliva as well as pancreatic and intestinal juices, is responsible for breaking down carbohydrates. Specific types of sugar also are broken down by amylase enzymes. Lactase breaks down milk sugar (lactose), for example, while maltase breaks down malt sugar (maltose), and sucrase breaks down cane and beet sugars (sucrose). The remaining digestive enzymes, protease and lipase, are responsible for protein and fat digestion.

In addition to the enzymes manufactured by the human body, they also can be found in certain raw foods, such as avocados, papayas, pineapples and bananas. Sprouts, however, provide the richest source of enzymes. Eating these enzyme-rich foods or, alternatively, taking enzyme supplements, will help prevent the depletion of the body's own enzymes, therefore reducing stress on the body.

All forms of enzymes should be kept in a cool place in order to ensure potency. Although powders and capsules should not be refrigerated because of their susceptibility to moisture, tablets and liquids may be stored in the icebox.

NOTE: Diabetic patients must consult with a qualified health care provider before adding any supplements to their daily regime. An appropriate provider would include an M.D., a registered dietitian, a nurse or pharmacist—but not a "nutritionist" with no accredited health training, or someone who sells supplements as a primary form of income.

12

Tips for Purchasing and Cooking Food

Purchasing fresh foods

It is important to purchase fruits, vegetables, fish, chicken and meats at their freshest. Here are some hints about how to purchase your foods and what to look for.

Vegetables

Avocado

Avocados will be soft and ready to eat in three to five days. Avoid mushy avocados with black spots.

Celery

For crisp, tender celery, avoid yellow leaves or woody stalks. Green Pascal is less stringy and more flavorful than the paler Golden Self-Blanching.

Lettuce

Lettuce should smell sweet, not bitter, and be free of brown edges. The greener your lettuce, the tastier your salads. Iceberg has the least amount of nutrients, and romaine lettuce has the most.

Onions
The skin of onions should be paper-dry, bright and satiny—so buying them loose from a bin gives you the best selection. Avoid onions that have sprouted or have soggy stem ends.

Potatoes
The best-quality potatoes are U.S. No. 1 Grade. Long, oval Idahoes are ideal for baking; red "new" potatoes are great boiled.

Seeds
The freshest seeds are sold in airtight packages. Keep them tightly sealed to prevent them from going bad (rancid).

Zucchini
A small- or medium-sized zucchini is the best. The skin should be smooth. Use at once, since it decays quickly.

Fruits

Bananas
A tinge of green at the stem, along with the scattered flecks of brown, show that they will be perfectly ripe and sweet in a day or so.

Papaya
A papaya one-third speckled with yellow will ripen in two days.

Pears
Pears are sold slightly underripe. Buy blemish-free fruit and let it sit on top of the refrigerator for a couple of days.

Pineapple
No soft spots or brown leaves. Leaves in the middle should come out easily.

Meats, poultry and fish

Roast

A well-marbled cut of meat makes a tender, juicy roast, but leaner cuts like top round would be a better choice. Moist cooking methods help retain flavor.

Chicken

Look for a plump, thick-skinned chicken. Yellow skin is no guarantee of freshness; it only means the bird has been fed corn.

Fish

Whole fish doesn't dry out as quickly as fillets or steaks. Look for bright, bulging eyes, tight, shiny scales and firm, translucent flesh and no "fishy" smell. Reject fish with dull-looking flesh or a limp, mushy look.

Dairy products

Cheese

Natural cheeses like Edam are much tastier and generally have fewer additives than processed cheese. However, be sure to trim away dyed wax or other outer coatings.

Eggs

Brown eggs are as nutritious as white. If there are any cracks, discard the egg.

Flavoring with herbs and spices

Using herbs and spices is a great way to enhance the flavor of your foods. It is the key to cooking wonderful meals. I use herbs and spices on meats, poultry, sauces, soups, vegetables and casseroles.

Below is a list of some spices I use. Try them; I know you will enjoy the taste of them.

All-Purpose Table Shake Seasoning
Replace the salt in your diet with Table Shake, a specially blended flavor that will perk up the flavors of your favorite foods without salt. It tastes great on vegetables, salads, poultry, fish, hamburgers and pork. Add to potatoes, pasta, rice, casseroles, soups and eggs. You can use it in place of salt when cooking or sprinkle it on foods served at the table.

Basil
Basil, also known as "sweet basil," is grown in the United States. You can sprinkle some on pizza or add it to salad dressings, tomato sauce, potatoes, eggplant, carrots, cauliflower and yellow squash. Use it to season vegetables and lentil soups. Melt some butter and brush the butter and basil on fish and scallops. It is also good with chicken or veal. Toss a little on your pasta; it tastes great!

Bay Leaves
Bay leaves are green and oblong. Add them to liquids when you are preparing pot roast, stews, vegetables, soups, spaghetti sauce and seafood chowders. When soups with bay leaves in them are simmering, there will be a wonderful aroma in your home.

Celery Salt
Celery salt is great in tomato juice. Add to salad dressing, coleslaw, chicken, potatoes and macaroni salad.

Chili Powder
Chili powder can be used in tomato juice, Spanish rice, soups and barbecue dishes. Add to Mexican-style dishes, such as enchiladas, tacos, refried beans and bean dip. Try sprinkling a little on your garlic bread.

Chives (Freeze-Dried)

Chives are hollow, reed-like stems of a plant in the allium family. Freeze-dried chives are preserved to hold their mild onion flavor and their beautiful green color. They're great to use in dips, sauces and salads, or to sprinkle on cottage cheese, yogurt and baked potatoes.

Ground Cinnamon

Cinnamon is such a wonderful flavor to add to hot cereal, puddings, waffle mix and pancake mix. Sprinkle some on your hot toast with a little butter. Also, use on ham, carrots and apples.

Cloves

Cloves are used on ham, soups, sauces, baked beans, biscuits, desserts, carrots and squash.

Cumin

Cumin is sold in both seed and ground forms. To get a different flavor for scrambled eggs or omelets, sprinkle cumin on them. Also, use cumin on meatloaf and chili.

Everglades Seasoning

This seasoning enhances the flavor of all different types of poultry and fish. You can sprinkle some on salads, vegetables, soups and even bread. This product does have a little sugar, but it is the next to the last ingredient.

Garlic

Garlic is absolutely wonderful. You can purchase it in cloves, garlic powder or garlic salt. Use in sauces, pizzas, stir fry, stews, meats, chicken, potatoes and breads. Eat some garlic, raw or cooked, for your health. It boosts the immune responses, helps lower blood pressure and cholesterol, and ranks very high in anti-cancer activity.

Ginger

Ginger has aromatic sweetness. It was one of the first oriental spices known to Europeans. Its hot, spicy-sweet flavor is used in cooking gingerbread, apple pie, cookies, cakes, fruits, carrots, yellow vegetables, soups, dressings and sweet potatoes.

Italian Seasoning

Italian Seasoning contains marjoram, thyme, rosemary, savory, sage, oregano and basil. This seasoning is excellent on pizza, tomato sauce, lasagna, manicotti, minestrone and spaghetti sauce. No kitchen should be without this seasoning.

Lemon Pepper

Want to spice up your boneless chicken, fish, shrimp, vegetables, cottage cheese and tomato salad? Sprinkle some lemon pepper in your tomato juice and turn it into a special beverage.

Marjoram

Marjoram is a grey-green herb in the mint family with a very pleasant spicy flavor. A lot of seasonings have marjoram in them. Use it in soups or stuffing mixtures for poultry or fish. Rub a little on meat or chicken before cooking.

Nutmeg

Nutmeg is a wonderful spice for spice cakes, fruit cakes, cookies and puddings. It's also good with carrots, spinach, sweet potatoes and mushroom soup. Add about ½ teaspoon of nutmeg to 1 cup of your favorite pancake mix, and your breakfast will taste so good.

Oregano

You can purchase oregano in leaf or ground form. This herb is mostly used in Italian dishes such as spaghetti sauce, pizza and lasagna.

Parsley

If you would like to add a sweet, somewhat spicy flavor to almost any food, then add a little parsley to it. Use it in soups, vegetable dishes, salad dressings and pasta. Stir parsley into melted garlic butter and spread over bread. Then broil the bread for a minute or so. You will have the best tasting garlic bread on earth.

Ethnic Seasonings

Mexican-American Seasonings

Mexican cooking in the United States relies heavily on the use of red or green salsa, which is made up of diced tomatoes, chilies, and onion. A typical combination of spices for meat dishes is dried oregano, ground cumin, and ground cloves. Cinnamon and bay leaves are also used. Cilantro, or fresh coriander, provides a distinctive taste in salsa, salads, and a wide variety of dishes. Chorizo, or ground pork sausage, is used to flavor dishes such as eggs, beans, and potatoes. This practice and the use of lard in cooking can make some dishes high in saturated fat. In addition, lemon juice, salt and pepper are popular seasonings for grilled meat.

Soul and Traditional Southern Seasonings

Fat in the form of fatback, salt port, bacon and ham hocks are used to flavor many Southern dishes. Vegetables, particularly greens, are boiled or stewed with water, fat and sometimes sugar. Sweet potatoes are baked in a syrup of butter, sugar, and spices such as cinnamon and nutmeg. Pickles and relishes made with sugar, salt and pepper are popular condiments. Meats, particularly pork and chicken, can be fried or grilled with barbecue sauce seasoned with red and black pepper. Using turkey bacon or ham, imitation bacon bits, or ham hocks with the fat removed can modify the fat content of many dishes. Recipes for delicious Southern desserts such as pound cake and pecan pie can be "lightened" to reduce the fat and sugar content.

Helpful cooking tips

Below is a list of different baking hints. I love to cook, and I have learned these different hints over the years. They have made a great difference in my cooking.

- When you are cooking a baked potato, pierce the skin with a fork to allow the steam to escape.

- When frying foods, remember that lard, margarine, and butter will burn before reaching the right temperature.

- When you are cooking meats, grill or broil them to lessen the fat content.

- When you are cutting meat or poultry, divide it into the same size pieces to assure that they will be cooked in the same amount of time.

- If you use glass or Corning Ware, reduce your conventional oven temperature by 25 degrees.

- If you do not want the baking dish cover to touch the top of your baked goods, insert toothpicks all over the top of the food item before putting the cover on.

- When you are preparing waffles, use buttermilk and just a pinch of baking soda instead of whole milk to make your waffles fluffy and light.

- If you have leftover waffle batter, add some finely chopped spinach to it for a vitamin-rich lunch or dinner waffle.

- When you are eating fruits and vegetables, eat the skin because it contains at least 10 percent of the entire nutritional content.

- Cook rice with beef, chicken or vegetable broth instead of water.

- When you boil pasta, add one tablespoon of oil to the water so that it does not boil over.

- When cooking vegetables, use a small amount of water. Avoid butter, oil, cream or cheeses as they are high in fat.

- If you want your eggs smoothly sliced, dip the knife in water first.

- If you want great scrambled eggs, make sure the eggs are not below room temperature.

- When you want to cut fat from your diet and add more flavor to your foods, use herbs and spices instead of butter.

- When cooking your poultry or meats for stews or soups, allow it to cool so that the fat can rise to the top and you can skim it off.

- When purchasing ground meat, choose only the leanest ground beef, pork and turkey—no more than 15 percent fat.

- Yellow-skinned onions are milder than white-skinned onions.

- For milder onions in your salad, try soaking the sliced pieces in milk first.

- When preparing vegetables, add a few slices of garlic to the cooking water to add a subtle flavor enhancement.

- When you want to remove the smell of onions from your hands, rub them with lemon juice and salt or vinegar.

- When cooking onions and garlic, use low to medium heat to prevent a bitter taste.

- When slow-cooking or roasting, use garlic to sweeten the flavor.

- Thoroughly cook all food of animal origin, including eggs. Cook meat to an internal temperature of 160 degrees, poultry to 180 degrees and fish to 160 degrees or until it is white and flaky.

Secrets to making great shakes and smoothies

- The blender canister should be set into the apparatus snugly and the top should be on tightly. I once blew the lid off my blender making a strawberry shake. The counter and walls were covered with strawberry juice!

- Add frozen fruit instead of a lot of ice. This will not only give you more vitamins and minerals, but it will make the smoothies extra refreshing.

- Tangy taste adds to a wonderful smoothie, so try adding yogurt, citrus juices, or a squirt of lemon or lime.

- Over-blending can make a smoothie too thick to drink. When using protein powder, add it last and blend until the powder disappears. If the shake or smoothie becomes too thick, add either ice cubes or a little cold water. Sometimes we like to make our smoothies thick so we can eat them like ice cream.

FOOD SUBSTITUTION LIST

INGREDIENTS ASKED FOR:	SUBSTITUTES:
1 teaspoon baking powder	½ teaspoon cream of tartar and ¼ teaspoon baking soda
1 tablespoon cornstarch	2 tablespoons flour
1 cup cake flour	1 cup all-purpose flour less 2 tablespoons
1 cup self-rising flour	1 cup all-purpose flour plus 1 teaspoon baking powder and ½ teaspoon salt
1 square (1 oz.) chocolate	3 tablespoons cocoa and 1 tablespoon butter
1 whole egg	2 egg yolks
2 large eggs	3 small eggs
1 cup buttermilk	1 cup milk and 1 tablespoon vinegar
1 cup milk	1 cup buttermilk and ½ teaspoon baking soda

FOOD EQUIVALENCIES

FOOD ITEM:	EQUIVALENT MEASURE:
1 medium apple	¾ cup chopped
1 medium banana	⅓ cup mashed
1 lemon peel, grated	1 teaspoon grated peel
1 medium lemon	3 tablespoons juice
1 medium lime	2 tablespoons juice
juice from 1 orange	6 to 7 tablespoons
1 orange peel, grated	2 teaspoons grated peel
1 medium orange	⅓ cup juice or 4 teaspoons shredded orange peel
1 medium pear	½ cup sliced
2 cups strawberries	1 cup puree
4 to 5 medium carrots	2 cups diced
1 medium onion	½ cup chopped
1 medium potato	½ cup mashed
1 large sweet potato	1½ cups diced
1 lb. large dried beans	2 cups uncooked
2 egg whites	1 whole egg
8 oz. macaroni	4 cups cooked
2 oz. spaghetti	1 cup cooked
1 cup uncooked rice	3 cups cooked
24 saltine crackers	1 cup fine crumbs
13 graham crackers	1 cup fine crumbs
22 vanilla wafers	1 cup crumbs
1 soft slice of bread	¾ cup soft crumbs
1 dry slice of bread	⅓ cup crumbs

FOOD ITEM:	EQUIVALENT MEASURE:
1 lb. walnuts or pecans	$4\frac{1}{2}$ cups
$\frac{1}{4}$ lb. chopped walnuts	1 cup
1 lb. almonds or peanuts	$3\frac{1}{4}$ cups
1 lb. cottage cheese	2 cups

13

Recipes

IN THIS CHAPTER ARE RECIPES for beverages, snacks, fun foods, breakfasts, lunches and dinners. Every one of these recipes is great for your entire family!

The number of servings each recipe will make and the approximate carbohydrate count per serving are included to help you with a daily food plan.

Juice drinks (no sugar added)

Apple-strawberry juice

1   cup strawberries
3   medium apples
½   cup water

Wash all fruit. Cut up to fit into juicer. Juice each fruit, add water and serve over ice.

Approximately 2 servings, 37 carbohydrates per serving

Strawberry-grape juice

12 medium strawberries
1   cup green grapes (seedless)
1   cup red grapes (seedless)
½   cup water

Wash all fruit. Cut up to fit into juicer. Juice each fruit, add water and serve over ice.

Approximately 3 servings, 26 carbohydrates per serving

Pineapple-strawberry-apple juice

10 medium strawberries
1   medium apple (peeled & cut)
1   round slice (1-inch thick) pineapple
¼   cup water

Wash all fruit. Cut up to fit into juicer. Juice each fruit, add water and serve over ice.

Approximately 2 servings, 23 carbohydrates per serving

Strawberry-apple-orange juice

1   cup strawberries
2   medium apples
2   oranges (peeled)
¼   cup water

Wash all fruit. Cut up to fit into juicer. Juice each fruit, add water and serve over ice.

Approximately 3 servings, 28 carbohydrates per serving

Strawberry-apple-kiwi juice

1   cup strawberries
2   kiwis (peeled)
3   small to medium apples
½   cup water

Wash all fruit. Cut up to fit into juicer. Juice each fruit, add water and serve over ice.

Approximately: 2½ servings, 37 carbohydrates per serving

Orange-kiwi-grape juice

1   cup red grapes (seedless)
3   kiwis (peeled)
1   orange (peeled)
¼   cup water

Wash all fruit. Cut up to fit into juicer. Juice each fruit, add water and serve over ice.

Approximately 2 servings, 38 carbohydrates per serving

Blueberry-apple juice

2   cups blueberries
2   medium apples
½   cup water

Wash all fruit. Cut up to fit into juicer. Juice each fruit, add water and serve over ice.

Approximately 2 servings, 34 carbohydrates per serving

Orange-lime juice

1   orange (peeled)
½   lime with the skin
½   cup sparkling mineral water, chilled
      crushed ice

Wash all fruit. Cut up to fit into juicer. Juice each fruit. In a food processor chop up enough ice to fill glass. Pour juice and mineral water over crushed ice.

Approximately 1 serving, 22 carbohydrates per serving

Watermelon juice

13   oz. watermelon
2   cups crushed ice

Wash fruit. Cut watermelon into small slices, keeping the rind on each slice. Put each slice into juicer. Chop up some ice in a food processor and pour melon juice over the cup of ice.

Approximately 1 serving, 13 carbohydrates per serving

Carrot-apple juice

6   medium carrots (cut tops off)
1   apple
2   tablespoons lemon juice

Wash all produce. Place the first two ingredients in juicer. Pour over a glass of ice, add lemon juice and serve immediately.

Approximately 2 servings, 34 carbohydrates per serving

Carrot-parsley-apple juice

7 medium carrots (cut tops off)
½ cup fresh parsley
3 apples
3 tablespoons lemon juice

Wash all produce. Place the first three ingredients in juicer. Pour over a glass of ice, add lemon juice and serve immediately.

Approximately 3 servings, 38 carbohydrates per serving

Carrot-parsley juice

5 medium carrots
5 sprigs of parsley
1 tablespoon lemon juice

Wash all produce. Place the first two ingredients in juicer. Pour over a glass of ice, add lemon juice and mix well.

Approximately 2 servings, 21 carbohydrates per serving

Lemonade

1 lemon
4 apples

Wash fruit. Place in juicer, process well. Serve over ice.

Approximately 2 servings, 38 carbohydrates per serving

Tasty Diet Sprite

1   can Diet Sprite
1   cup strawberries (frozen or fresh)

Wash fruit. Combine Diet Sprite and strawberries in blender. Blend on medium speed until smooth. Serve over ice.

Approximately 3 servings, 5 carbohydrates per serving

Banana lemonade

1   medium banana (peeled)
1   medium lemon (peeled)
1   cup pineapple juice (unsweetened)
½   cup ice water
1   cup ice cubes

Combine all the ingredients in blender. Blend on high speed until smooth. Serve over ice.

Approximately 3 servings, 18 carbohydrates per serving

Smoothies

Strawberry-banana juice smoothie

1   cup strawberries
2   medium bananas (peeled)
¾   cup soy milk
2   tablespoons instant powdered milk
1   teaspoon lemon juice
½   cup ice cubes

Combine all ingredients in blender. Blend on medium speed until smooth and serve.

Approximately 3 servings, 21 carbohydrates per serving

Pineapple fruit smoothie

1   cup pineapple (in unsweetened pineapple juice)
2   small bananas (peeled)
1   cup frozen strawberries
1   tablespoon protein powder
½   cup soy or rice milk
½   cup ice

Combine all ingredients in blender. Blend on medium speed until smooth and serve.

Approximately 3½ servings, 26 carbohydrates per serving

Banana-pineapple juice smoothie

2   medium bananas (peeled)
1   cup crushed pineapple
½   cup plain yogurt
¼   cup soy or rice milk
1   tablespoon protein powder
1   cup ice

Combine all ingredients in blender. Blend on high speed until smooth and serve.

Approximately 3 servings, 30 carbohydrates per serving

Summer breeze smoothie

1   cup plain yogurt
1   medium banana (peeled)
1   cup frozen strawberries
1   medium kiwi (peeled)
1   cup water
1   cup ice
1   tablespoon protein powder

Combine all ingredients in blender. Blend on medium speed until smooth and serve.

Approximately 4 servings, 16 carbohydrates per serving

Honeydew-cantaloupe smoothie

¾   cup honeydew (peeled)
½   cup cantaloupe (peeled)
1   cup frozen strawberries
2   cups water
3   teaspoons lime juice
1   cup ice cubes

Combine all ingredients in blender. Blend on medium speed until smooth and serve.

Approximately 5 servings, 9 carbohydrates per serving

Tangerine bash smoothie

1   small banana (peeled)
1   cup strawberries
2   medium tangerines (peeled)
1   cup ice cubes

½   cup water
1   tablespoon protein powder
1   tablespoon instant powdered milk

Combine all ingredients in blender. Blend on high speed until smooth and serve. If the smoothie becomes too thick, add a little water.

Approximately 4 servings, 15 carbohydrates per serving

Shakes

Fruity shake

1   cup grapes (seedless)
1   medium apple (peeled and sliced)
½   cup orange juice
½   cup frozen strawberries
½   cup low-fat milk or soy milk
½   cup sugar-free frozen strawberry ice cream
1   tablespoon protein powder

Combine all ingredients in blender. Blend on high speed until smooth and serve.

Approximately 4 servings, 23 carbohydrates per serving

Banana-strawberry energy shake

2   bananas (peeled)
1   cup strawberries
¾   cup plain non-fat yogurt
¼   cup vanilla low-fat light yogurt
1   cup soy milk

1   teaspoon vanilla extract
8   ice cubes
pinch of cinnamon

Combine bananas, strawberries, skim milk and ice cubes in blender. Blend until smooth. Add yogurts, vanilla extract and cinnamon. Blend on medium speed until well blended and serve. If the shake becomes too thick, add a little water.

Approximately 3½ servings, 26 carbohydrates per serving

Strawberry delight shake

1   cup low–fat plain yogurt
½   cup soy milk
2   cups strawberries
1   medium pear (peeled)
1   medium green apple (peeled)
10   ice cubes

Combine all ingredients in blender in the order listed. Blend on medium speed until smooth. Serve with a couple of strawberries on the side.

Approximately 4 servings, 24 carbohydrates per serving

Cool afternoon shake

1   cup grapes (seedless)
1   medium banana (peeled)
10   strawberries
¼   cup soy milk
¼   cup no-sugar-added vanilla ice cream
1   tablespoon protein powder
1   ice cube

Combine all ingredients in blender. Blend on high speed until smooth and serve.

Approximately 4 servings, 17 carbohydrates per serving

Tangerine fruit shake

1	medium tangerine (peeled)
1	cup plain yogurt
1	medium banana (peeled)
1	cup strawberries
2	cups ice cubes
½	cup water
1	tablespoon strawberry protein powder

Combine all ingredients in blender in the order listed. Blend on medium speed until smooth and serve.

Approximately 4½ servings, 14 carbohydrates per serving

Fun foods

Fruity pops

My little girl gave this treat its name. She loves frozen fruits in the summertime.

1	pint strawberries (or any fruit of your choice)
6	popsicle sticks
2	small ziploc freezer bags

Poke a popsicle stick through 3 whole strawberries. Four Fruity Pops will fit into 1 small ziploc bag. Place Fruity Pops in freezer for at least 6 hours. They will keep for about about a month.

Approximately 6 servings, 5 carbohydrates per serving

Frozen yogurt pops

My son loves frozen yogurt. I make the pops at home so that I know exactly what he is eating. This is a wonderful snack for everyone!

     8 oz. fat-free plain yogurt
1    $4\frac{1}{2}$-oz. can of diced peaches (or any fruit of your choice, no sugar added)
2   popsicle sticks

Remove approximately 2 full teaspoons of yogurt from the carton and discard. Add fruit to yogurt and mix well. Make two slits in the middle of the lid with a sharp knife, $\frac{1}{4}$-inch apart. Insert one popsicle stick into each slit. Place in freezer overnight.

Approximately 1 serving, 32 carbohydrates per serving

Candy popcorn balls

Candy popcorn balls are a favorite among the children in our neighborhood.

10   cups popped popcorn
$\frac{1}{2}$ cup sugar-free taffy, any flavor
$\frac{1}{4}$ cup margarine
1   cup peanuts
1   box strawberry sugar-free Jello (or any flavor of your choice)

Pour popped popcorn and peanuts into a large bowl and set aside. Cut taffy into small pieces and set aside. Microwave margarine in a bowl on high for about 30 seconds. Remove margarine from microwave and add all the taffy. Microwave margarine and taffy on high for 1 minute. Remove bowl and mix with spoon. Add Jello to taffy mixture; stir mixture well. Pour taffy mixture over popcorn and peanuts. Quickly stir with spoon until taffy mixture evenly coats the popcorn and peanuts.

Grease your hands well with margarine. Shape mixture into balls. Allow balls to cool completely on waxed paper.

Approximately 18 servings, 7 carbohydrates per servings

Striped Jello parfait

This is very colorful and makes a great dessert on a hot summer day.

1 box strawberry or cherry sugar-free Jello
1 box lime sugar-free Jello
½ cup plain yogurt
½ cup light Cool Whip
   cherries or strawberries

Combine lime Jello and 1 cup boiling water in a bowl; stir until Jello dissolves. Add 1 cup of cold water and stir. Divide evenly into 6 parfait cups and refrigerate for about 1 hour or until gelatin is thick.

Add 1 cup of boiling water to cherry Jello in a separate bowl and stir until Jello dissolves. Add 1 cup of cold water and stir. Allow to stand at room temperature for 10 minutes. Pour an even amount of cherry Jello into each parfait cup over each layer of lime Jello. Chill for about 4 hours or until it jiggles. Top with Cool Whip and cherries or strawberries.

Approximately 6 servings, 3 carbohydrates per servings

Taffy crispy treats

These are the best tasting crispy treats, and no sugar has been added. These are great for any party.

    4   tablespoons butter or margarine
    22 sugar-free taffy candies (strawberry, orange, vanilla or mixed)
    5   cups Rice Krispies

Spray a 13" x 9" x 2" baking pan with a non-stick coating. Melt butter in a saucepan over low heat. Add taffy, stirring constantly until completely melted. Remove from heat and quickly add Rice Krispies, stirring until all pieces are evenly coated. Butter a spoon and press the Rice Krispies into the pan. Allow to cool for about 1½ hours. Cut into 24 squares.

Approximately 24 servings, 10 carbohydrates per serving

Yogurt-applesauce snack

This dish can be served as a side dish or a quick snack.

    ½   cup low-fat plain light yogurt
    ½   cup low-fat vanilla light yogurt
    1   cup unsweetened applesauce

Combine yogurts, then add applesauce. Mix well.

Approximately 4 servings, 13 carbohydrates per serving

Cookie banana stick

Cookie banana sticks are nutritious snacks and so much fun to eat!

1   medium banana
4   small butter cookies
2   popsicle sticks

Cut banana in half. Crumble cookies. Insert popsicle sticks into banana halves. Place a couple of drops of water on each banana half, and roll bananas in the cookie crumbs. Place in separate small ziploc bags and freeze.

Approximately 2 servings, 14 carbohydrates per serving

Carrot-pineapple cup

Carrots and pineapples are so good that we decided to put them together for a mid-afternoon snack. This dish also makes a wonderful dessert after a hot meal.

1   cup grated carrot
½   cup unsweetened crushed pineapple

Combine grated carrots and pineapple.

Approximately 3 servings, 18 carbohydrates per serving

Baggy mix

This snack is healthy and portable. The kids like to take a bag with them when they are playing in the tree house.

1   cup Wheat Chex
1   cup Cheerios
2   cups low-fat microwave popcorn
1   cup miniature pretzels, fat-free
½   cup raisins

Mix all ingredients together. Divide into 6 small locking plastic snack bags for portability, or store in an air-tight container.

Approximately 6 servings, 28 carbohydrates per serving

Sweet and spicy popcorn

When you want something spicy and something sweet at the same time, try this great recipe.

¾   cup uncooked popcorn
¼   cup melted butter
1   teaspoon salt
¾   teaspoon garlic powder
1¼   teaspoon cayenne pepper
¾   teaspoon cumin
¾   cup raisins
1   cup honey-roasted peanuts

Pop popcorn according to the package directions. Pour popcorn into a large bowl, set aside. In a small bowl combine the next five ingredients and pour over popcorn. Mix well. Stir in peanuts and raisins.

Approximately 15 servings, 16 carbohydrates per serving

Pudding cream puffs

I made this treat for Christmas one year and everyone raved over it. They could not believe it was a sugar-free dessert. Now it's a Christmas tradition in our home.

½   cup butter (1 stick)
1   cup water
1   cup flour
4   eggs
    confectioners sugar or sugar-free chocolate (optional)
    vanilla pudding (recipe below)

Preheat oven to 400 degrees. In medium saucepan, add butter and water, bring to a boil. Remove pan from burner. Add flour and mix. Add eggs to flour mixture and stir for about 2 minutes until the dough is soft. Using a large tablespoon, drop dough onto ungreased cookie sheet, leaving about three inches between drops. Bake for 30 to 35 minutes. Remove from oven and allow to cool.

Poke a hole into the side of each puff and fill puffs with sugar-free vanilla pudding. Sprinkle the top with a little confectioners sugar or spread a little sugar-free chocolate fudge on top. Store pudding cream puffs in the refrigerator.

Approximately 10 servings, 13 carbohydrates per serving

Vanilla pudding (cream puff filling)

2   1-oz. boxes sugar-free vanilla pudding
3   cups skim milk

Pour boxes of vanilla pudding into a bowl. Add cold skim milk and beat well with a wire whisk.

Approximately 12 servings, 12 carbohydrates

Sweet potato chips

Everyone loves potato chips, and the whole family will go crazy over sweet potato chips.

2   large sweet potatoes (peeled and sliced ⅛-inch thick)
1½ teaspoons olive oil
¼   teaspoon chili powder
    pinch of salt

Dip:

1   cup plain non-fat yogurt
1   clove garlic (minced)
½   teaspoon ground cumin
¼   teaspoon freshly ground black pepper

Preheat oven to 400 degrees. While oven is heating, blend dip ingredients in a bowl and chill. In a separate bowl, toss potatoes, oil, chili powder and salt. Place potatoes on non-stick baking sheet. Bake until golden (20 to 25 minutes). Turn and bake for 10 more minutes. Cool on wire rack.

Approximately 4 servings, 28 carbohydrates per serving

Pudding pie

Family and friends always ask me to make this pie on holidays.

1   graham cracker pie shell
1   2.1-oz. package sugar-free instant chocolate pudding
1   2.1-oz. package sugar-free instant vanilla pudding
1   4-oz. package light cream cheese
1   3-oz. container fat-free Cool Whip
1   teaspoon vanilla extract

⅓ cup confectioners sugar
3 cups skim milk
2 plain graham crackers

In a bowl, combine chocolate and vanilla pudding with milk. Mix well with a whisk. Pour mixture into pie shell. Combine cream cheese, sugar and vanilla extract in a separate bowl; mix well. Fold Cool Whip into cream cheese mixture, and pour on top of pie.

Crumble graham crackers over pie. Place in freezer for about one hour, then move to refrigerator for 30 minutes before serving.

Approximately 6 servings, 37 carbohydrates per serving

Frozen strawberry pie

4 cups sugar-free strawberry frozen yogurt or ice cream
1 6-oz. container fat-free Cool Whip
1 9-inch ready made pie crust
   fresh strawberries (optional)

Thaw Cool Whip in refrigerator. Thaw yogurt or ice cream just enough so that it can be stirred into the Cool Whip. (Do not allow it to become too soft.) Mix well and spread mixture in pie crust. Freeze. Before serving, add fresh strawberries to top.

Approximately 6 servings, 30 carbohydrates per serving

Fruit dish

This fruit dish is a refreshing treat on a hot summer day.

⅓ cup plain non-fat yogurt
⅓ cup light sour cream

½ teaspoon vanilla extract
1 teaspoon firmly packed light brown sugar
1 cup fresh strawberries
1 cup seedless grapes
1 tablespoon salted peanuts, crushed

Wash fruit. Mix the first four ingredients in a large bowl. Add fruit and mix well. Cover and chill for about two hours. When ready to serve, pour evenly into 3 parfait glasses, and top with crushed peanuts.

Approximately 3 servings, 30 carbohydrates

Breakfast

Breakfast delight
4 slices pineapple
1 banana
2 cups soy milk
3 tablespoons protein powder
1 tablespoon honey

Combine all ingredients in blender. Blend well and serve.

Approximately 4 servings, 28 carbohydrates per serving

Cinnamon heart-shaped French toast
Everyone loves French toast. Your kids will want to help you make this pretty variation.

2 eggs
¼ teaspoon cinnamon

½   teaspoon vanilla extract
1   teaspoon sugar
6   slices white bread
    dash of nutmeg
1   heart-shaped cookie cutter (medium to large)
    strawberries (optional)

Combine all ingredients except bread and strawberries in a medium bowl. Mix well. Lightly spray frying pan with vegetable spray. Preheat stove to 350 degrees. Place the cookie cutter on top of one slice of bread at a time, and cut out heart shapes. Discard excess bread. Dip one slice of bread at a time into the egg mixture. Coat well. Brown bread on both sides and serve with a couple of strawberries on top.

Approximately 3 servings, 23 carbohydrates per serving

Breakfast cheese toast

If you can't get your children to eat, try this cheese toast. It's worked for us every time.

4   slices wheat bread
4   slices light American cheese
    butter

Spread some butter on the bread and place each piece on a cookie sheet. Put a slice of cheese on top of buttered bread. Bake at 350 degrees for about 3 minutes or until cheese is melted.

Approximately 2 servings, 22 carbohydrates per serving

Tasty fruity oatmeal

Breakfast is an important meal, and this fruity oatmeal has everything you need to start the day. Just add a glass of homemade juice and you're on your way to a great day!

- ¾ cup water
- ½ cup soy or skim milk
- ½ teaspoon cinnamon
- ½ cup rolled oats
- ½ cup chopped apple (peeled)
- 2 tablespoons raisins
- ½ teaspoon brown sugar

In a medium saucepan, bring milk and water almost to a boil. Add rolled oats, cinnamon and apples. Cook uncovered for about five minutes or until the liquid is absorbed. Add raisins and brown sugar and serve.

Approximately 2 servings, 33 carbohydrates per serving

Cinnamon toast

A little cinnamon toast with your breakfast gets you ready to start a new day.

- 2 slices white bread
- ⅓ cup low-fat cottage cheese
- ⅓ teaspoon sugar
- ⅓ teaspoon cinnamon

Toast bread until golden. Spread cottage cheese on top, sprinkle with sugar and cinnamon. Place on a cookie sheet and broil just long enough for the topping to bubble. Serve immediately.

Approximately 2 servings, 15 carbohydrates per serving

Applesauce waffles

My children love to help me prepare breakfast. This recipe is easy and fun to make.

2   cups whole wheat flour
2   cups water
2   eggs
1   tablespoon olive oil or corn oil
½   teaspoon salt
3½   cups unsweetened applesauce
    strawberries and blackberries (optional)

Place all ingredients in a bowl and blend for about 2 minutes with an electric mixer. Spoon mixture into a hot waffle iron. Cook until golden brown. Serve hot. Top with strawberries and blackberries.

Approximately 6 servings, 26 carbohydrates per serving

Strawberry breakfast shake

This is what I make for my family in the mornings when we're in a hurry. Add a couple pieces of wheat toast for a complete breakfast.

1   envelope Knox unflavored gelatin
1   cup soy or skim milk
¼   cup low-fat cottage cheese
1   cup low-fat plain yogurt
2½   cups strawberries, sliced (fresh or frozen)

Place all ingredients in blender in the order listed above. Blend thoroughly. Serve immediately.

Approximately 4 servings, 18 carbohydrates per serving

Cinnamon roll toast

When we want something a little different to go with our eggs and fruit, we make these little cinnamon rolls.

1½   teaspoons cinnamon
1   tablespoon sugar
4   slices of white bread
1   tablespoon melted butter
2   tablespoons light cream cheese

Mix cinnamon and sugar together in a small bowl and set aside. Trim crust off bread and spread cream cheese on each slice. Roll up each slice of bread, then cut each of the rolls into thirds to make three little rolls. Turn each piece in butter to coat lightly, then roll them in cinnamon mixture. Bake on ungreased cookie sheet for about 12 minutes at 350 degrees.

Approximately 2 servings, 22 carbohydrates per serving

Banana mash pancakes

1   medium banana
1   egg
½   cup wheat flour
½   teaspoon vanilla extract
2   teaspoons baking powder
      fruit (optional)

Mash banana. Add egg and vanilla and mix. Add flour and baking powder, and mix well. Spray a frying pan with non-stick cooking spray. Cook over medium heat until bubbles form on top. Turn and cook until both sides are golden brown. Top with fruit. Serve hot.

Approximately 3 servings, 23 carbohydrates per serving

Lunch

Banana-peanut butter sandwich

Once you've eaten this sandwich, you'll always come back for more. The neighborhood children come over and for this treat along with a fruit juice.

- 4 slices raisin bread
- 1 medium banana (sliced)
- 4 tablespoons peanut butter

Slice banana lengthwise and cut into halves. Toast raisin bread. Spread peanut butter on toast and add banana slices on top. Serve warm.

Approximately 2 servings, 42 carbohydrates per serving

Spinach-tuna sandwich

- 1 6-oz. can of tuna (white, packed in water)
- 2 tablespoons light mayonnaise
- 1 teaspoon relish
- ⅓ cup fresh spinach (chopped)
- 2 slices bread

Mix the first four ingredients together in a small bowl. Toast bread if desired. Spread mixture between slices of bread. Eat and enjoy!

Approximately 1 serving, 22 carbohydrates per serving

Turkey spinach salad

Spinach is a wonderful source of beta-carotene and Vitamin A. This dish is healthy and tastes great.

1	package fresh spinach
1	cup turkey (cup up)
2	hard–boiled eggs (sliced)
1	tomato (cut up)
1	cucumber (sliced)
2	carrots (sliced)
¼	cup low-fat cheddar cheese (optional)

Rinse spinach. In a large bowl, mix all ingredients. Add your favorite salad dressing and toss well. Sprinkle with a little cheddar cheese if desired.

Approximately 4 servings, 15 carbohydrates per serving

Pizza muffin

These individual pizzas are perfect for an outside picnic under a shade tree.

1	English muffin (cut in half and toasted lightly)
4	teaspoons pizza sauce
½	cup shredded mozzarella cheese
6	pieces pepperoni

Spread 2 teaspoons of pizza sauce on each muffin. Sprinkle mozzarella cheese on top. Top with pepperoni. Broil until the cheese melts. Serve hot.

Approximately 1 serving, 28 carbohydrates per serving

Baked French fries

Truly the best fries in town!

3   large potatoes (not peeled)
1   tablespoon olive oil
2   teaspoons paprika
   salt

Preheat oven to 450 degrees. Slice potatoes about ¼-inch thick. Place in a 13" x 9" baking dish and sprinkle with oil and paprika. Toss so that the oil coats all potatoes. Bake for about 12 minutes. Turn potatoes with a spatula. Bake for about 25 to 28 minutes more, turning a couple of times. Sprinkle with salt and serve hot.

Approximately 4 servings, 30 carbohydrates per serving

Veggie dip

If you like dip, try this one.

1   cup plain non-fat yogurt
1   package Good Seasonings dry salad mix
   assorted vegetables, cut up

Combine yogurt and salad mix in a bowl. Mix well. Refrigerate for three to four hours. Serve with vegetables.

Approximately 4 servings, 5 carbohydrates per serving

Dinner

Pizza chicken

If you love pizza, try this nutritious and delicious recipe.

1   8-oz. jar spaghetti sauce
¼   cup Italian bread crumbs
6   pieces of chicken (breast or thighs)
1   8-oz. package low-fat mozzarella (shredded)

Toss chicken in bread crumbs until evenly coated. Place chicken in a shallow pan. Pour spaghetti sauce over it. Bake at 350 degrees for 45 minutes or until chicken is tender. Sprinkle mozzarella cheese over chicken. Cover and cook for at least 5 minutes.

Approximately 6 servings, 9 carbohydrates per serving

Old-fashioned spaghetti sauce

I always helped my mom make spaghetti sauce when I was young. To this day, I still make it the same way.

1   medium chopped onion
1   lb. lean hamburger or ground turkey
1   teaspoon garlic salt
2   tablespoons Italian seasoning
2   tablespoons oregano
½   teaspoon pepper
1   teaspoon salt
1   teaspoon sweet basil
1   28-oz. can tomato puree
½   cup water
1   teaspoon sugar
2   bay leaves

Sauté onion and meat. When meat is partially cooked, add garlic salt, Italian seasoning, oregano, pepper, salt and sweet basil. Continue to cook until well done. Drain and set aside. In a large cooking pan, pour in puree and water; add sugar and bay leaves. Add the meat to the sauce and mix well. Simmer on low for 3 hours or more. Stir a couple of times each hour. May be used immediately, or refrigerated or frozen.

Approximately 8 servings, 1 carbohydrate per serving

Cheese twist

Our children love noodles any way they're cooked. This recipe is a favorite at our church picnics.

1   package rotelli (corkscrew noodles), cooked as directed
2   cups shredded low-fat mozzarella cheese
   Old-fashioned spaghetti sauce

Make spaghetti sauce as directed in the previous recipe. Mix cooked noodles into prepared spaghetti sauce. Sprinkle shredded mozzarella cheese on top. Let simmer on very low heat for about 15 minutes. Mix well before serving.

Approximately 8 servings, 42 carbohydrates per serving

Fifteen-bean soup

This nutritious meal is convenient, too. It cooks in a crock pot all day, and when dinnertime comes, voilà! Your meal is ready to serve.

2   cups 15-bean soup mix (dry beans)
1   slice ham, center piece
1   medium onion (chopped)

1   cup celery (chopped)
½   cup carrots (sliced)
½   teaspoon salt
½   teaspoon pepper
½   teaspoon garlic salt
2   bay leaves
2   cups water
3   14–oz. cans chicken broth

Rinse beans. Soak them in 2 cups of water for about an hour. Drain. Trim fat from ham and cut into small pieces. Mix all ingredients together in the crock-pot. Stir well. Cook on high for about 3 to 4 hours or on low for about 11 hours. The beans will be tender when fully cooked.

Approximately 6 servings, 30 carbohydrates per serving

Spinach pie

This Greek favorite is so good that the kids never realize they're eating spinach!

1   9-inch pie shell, frozen
2   10-oz. package chopped spinach, thawed and drained
1   15-oz. package low-fat ricotta cheese
2   eggs
1   medium onion (chopped)
     salt, pepper, nutmeg to taste

Sauté onions in butter with a little salt, pepper and nutmeg. At the same time, bake pie shell at 400 degrees for about 2 minutes. Combine all ingredients and pour into pie shell. Bake at 375 degrees for about 50 to 60 minutes.

Approximately 6 servings, 24 carbohydrates per serving

Zucchini casserole

Zucchini casserole is a wonderful side dish. My children love it.

1   cup pancake mix (use a mix that requires the addition of water only)
3   medium zucchini
1   medium onion
1   lb. package low-fat cheddar cheese (shredded)

Mix pancake mix and water as directed on box. Keep batter a little thick. Set aside. Slice zucchini into round pieces. Slice onion into thin round slices. Dip zucchini into pancake batter and place a few slices across bottom of baking dish. Repeat with onion, and layer onion on top of zucchini. Sprinkle some cheese on top for another layer. Repeat. Bake at 350 degrees for 35 minutes.

Approximately 6 servings, 19 carbohydrates per serving

Fried rice

This is an old favorite of my great-great-grandmother, who loved to cook for everyone.

1   cup fine egg noodles, cooked
2   tablespoons olive oil
¾   cup minute rice
1   cup carrots (cooked and diced)
1   small can mushrooms
1   can beef consommé

Brown the noodles in olive oil. Add all other ingredients. Cover and simmer for 10 minutes or until rice is tender.

Approximately 5 servings, 23 carbohydrates per serving

Brown rice

1½ cups brown minute rice
2   cups chicken broth
½   cup shredded carrots
¼   cup peas

In a medium pot, bring rice and chicken broth to a boil. Cover and simmer for 10 minutes. Add carrots and peas, and simmer for about 5 more minutes. Serve hot.

Approximately 5 servings, 30 carbohydrates per serving

Cheesy potato casserole

My children love cheese and potatoes; they ask me to make this dish all the time.

3   cups mashed potatoes (made from 6 medium potatoes)
1   teaspoon salt
½   teaspoon pepper
1½ teaspoons cumin
½   cup low-fat cheddar cheese
3   eggs (beaten)
¼   cup grated cheese

Prepare mashed potatoes according to your favorite recipe. Add salt, pepper, cumin, cheddar cheese and eggs, and mix together well. Pour potato mixture into greased casserole dish. Top with grated cheese. Bake at 400 degrees for 18 minutes.

Approximately 4 servings, 26 carbohydrates per serving

Best baked potato ever

4 small baking potatoes
2 teaspoons olive oil
1 teaspoon salt
2 paper towels

Pierce potato skins all over with a fork to allow the steam to escape. Place potatoes on one paper towel in the microwave. Place a moist paper towel over potatoes. Microwave on high for 6 minutes. Turn potatoes over. Cook for 5 more minutes on high. Rub potatoes with olive oil, then with salt. Cook for another 2 minutes on high. Turn and cook 2 more minutes on high. Serve warm.

Approximately 4 servings, 15 carbohydrates per serving

Baked sweet potatoes

Sweet potatoes are a great source of vitamins.

4 sweet potatoes
1 tablespoon olive oil or corn oil

Preheat oven to 350 degrees. Wash and dry potatoes. Rub jackets with oil. Pierce potato skins all over with a fork to allow the steam to escape. Bake on a cookie sheet for 1 hour or until tender.

Approximately 4 servings, 28 carbohydrates per serving

Garlic cheese bread

This bread tastes great with any meal.

1   small loaf French bread
2½ tablespoons butter or margarine
1   teaspoon garlic powder
¼   cup grated parmesan cheese

With a bread knife, cut 7 deep slits diagonally across bread loaf, but do not cut all the way through. Spread butter in each slit, then sprinkle with garlic powder and parmesan cheese. Wrap loaf with foil and cook for 15 minutes at 350 degrees.

Approximately 8 servings, 15 carbohydrates per serving

Banana nut bread

This recipe makes a delicious dessert. For more of a treat, top it off with a scoop of sugar-free ice cream.

2   cups flour
2   teaspoons baking powder
½   teaspoon baking soda
½   teaspoon salt
¼   cup butter
¼   cup sugar
2   eggs
2   medium ripe bananas (mashed)
½   cup buttermilk
     nuts (optional)

Preheat oven to 350 degrees. Mix flour, baking powder, baking soda and salt in a bowl. In a separate bowl, cream butter and sugar together, then add eggs and bananas. Pour buttermilk and flour mixture alternately into a greased loaf pan. Bake for 1 hour.

Approximately 16 servings, 15 carbohydrates per serving

14

Diabetes Control and Complications Trial (DCCT)

THE DIABETES CONTROL AND Complications Trial (DCCT) is a clinical study that was conducted from 1983 to 1992 by the National Institute of Diabetes and Digestive and Kidney Diseases (NIDDK). The study showed that keeping blood sugar levels as close to normal as possible slows the onset and progression of eye, kidney, and nerve diseases caused by diabetes. In fact, it demonstrated that any sustained lowering of blood sugar helps, even if the person has a history of poor control.

The DCCT is the largest, most comprehensive diabetes study ever conducted. It involved 1,441 volunteers with insulin-dependent diabetes mellitus (Type 1) in 29 medical centers in the United States and Canada. Volunteers had diabetes for at least one year, but no longer than fifteen years. They also were required to have no, or only very early, signs of diabetic eye disease.

The study compared the effects of two treatment regimens: standard therapy and intensive control with the complications of diabetes. Volunteers were assigned to each treatment group randomly.

Intensive treatment

All DCCT participants were monitored for diabetic retinopathy, which typically affects people with long-standing, poorly controlled diabetes. The retina is the light-sensing tissue at the back of the eye. Study results showed that intensive therapy reduced the risk for developing retinopathy by 76 percent. In participants with some eye damage at the beginning of the study, intensive management slowed the progression of the disease by 54 percent.

According to the National Eye Institute, one branch of the National Institute of Health, as many as 24,000 persons with diabetes lose their sight each year. In the United States, diabetic retinopathy is the leading cause of blindness in adults under age 65.

Participants in the DCCT were tested to assess the development of diabetic kidney disease (nephropathy). Findings showed that intensive treatment prevented the development and slowed the progression of diabetic kidney disease by 50 percent.

Kidney disease from diabetes is the most common cause of kidney failure in the United States and the greatest threat to life in adults with Type 1 diabetes. Diabetes damages the small blood vessels in the kidneys, impairing their ability to filter impurities from blood for excretion in the urine. Persons with kidney damage must have a kidney transplant or rely on dialysis to cleanse their blood. After having diabetes for fifteen years, one-third of the people with Type 1 develop kidney disease.

Participants in the DCCT also were examined to detect the development of nerve damage (diabetic neuropathy). Study results showed the risk of nerve damage was reduced by 60 percent in persons undergoing intensive treatment.

Diabetic nerve disease can cause pain and loss of feeling in the feet, legs, and fingertips. It can also affect the parts of the nervous system that control blood pressure, heart rate, digestion, and sexual function. Neuropathy is a major contributing factor in foot and leg amputations among people with diabetes.

DCCT participants were not anticipated to have many heart-related problems because their average age was only 27 when the study began. Nevertheless, they underwent cardiograms, blood pressure tests and laboratory tests of blood fat levels to look for signs of cardiovascular disease. The study proved that volunteers undergoing intensive treatment had a significantly lower risk level for developing high blood cholesterol, which is a cause of heart disease. The risk was 35 percent lower in these volunteers, suggesting that intensive treatment can help prevent heart disease.

Elements of intensive management in the DCCT:

- Testing blood sugar levels four or more times a day
- Four daily insulin injections or use of insulin pump
- Adjustment of insulin doses according to food intake and exercise
- A diet and exercise plan
- Monthly visits to a health care team consisting of a physician, nurse educator, dietitian, and behavioral therapist

In the DCCT, the most significant side effect of intensive treatment was an increase in the risk for low blood sugar (hypoglycemia). Severe hypoglycemia episodes could require assistance from another person. Because of this risk, DCCT researchers do not recommend intensive therapy for children under age 13, people with heart disease or advanced complications, older adults, and people with a history of frequent severe hypoglycemia. Persons in the intensive management group also gained a modest amount of weight, suggesting that intensive treatment may not be appropriate for diabetics who are overweight.

DCCT researchers estimate that intensive management doubles the cost of managing diabetes because of increased visits to health care professionals and the need for more frequent blood testing at home. However, this cost is offset by the reduction in medical expenses related to long-term complications and by the improved quality of life of people with diabetes.

Summary of DCCT study

Lowering blood sugar reduces risk:

Eye disease	76% reduced risk
Kidney disease	50% reduced risk
Nerve disease	60% reduced risk
Cardiovascular disease	35% reduced risk

Diabetic retinopathy

Eye disease, or retinopathy, is the leading cause of blindness. It is caused by damage to the blood vessels of the retina. In some people with diabetes, retinal blood vessels may swell and leak fluid. In other people, abnormal new blood vessels grow on the surface of the retina, causing partial loss of vision or blindness.

In the beginning stages, there are no symptoms. Vision may not change until the disease becomes more severe. Also, it is usually painless.

Anyone with diabetes can get retinopathy. The longer one has diabetes, the more likely he or she is to develop retinopathy. Almost half of all the people with diabetes will develop some degree of diabetic retinopathy during their lifetimes. But with good control of diabetes, the number of cases of retinopathy will be reduced.

The American Diabetes Association (ADA) recommends testing all children with diabetes once they have had the disease for five or more years and have reached puberty. Examinations should be done on an annual basis, and more frequently if necessary. The eyes need to be dilated during the exam using eye drops to enlarge the pupils so the doctor can see more of the insides of the eyes to check for signs of disease.

Laser surgery is used to treat some cases of retinopathy. A strong beam of light is aimed into the retina to shrink the abnormal vessels. Laser surgery has been proven to reduce the risk of severe vision loss up to 90 percent. If one has already lost vision, laser surgery often cannot restore sight. But with early detection, it is often the best way to prevent vision loss caused by diabetes.

Retinopathy cannot be prevented totally, but the risks of getting the disease can be reduced greatly by keeping tight control of blood sugar levels. The DCCT proved that if one maintains close-to-normal blood sugar levels, there will be a lower frequency of eye, kidney and nerve disease.

15

Diabetes Research

THE FEDERAL GOVERNMENT and nongovernmental organizations such as the Juvenile Diabetes Foundation (JDF) and the American Diabetes Association (ADA) all support research to improve the health and well-being of people with diabetes and to find ways to prevent and cure the disease.

The National Institute of Diabetes and Digestive and Kidney Diseases (NIDDK) supports basic and clinical research in its own laboratories, in research centers and at hospitals throughout the United States. The NIDDK also gathers and analyzes statistics about diabetes. Other NIH branches carry out research on diabetes-related eye diseases, heart and vascular complications, pregnancy and dental problems. Other government agencies that sponsor diabetes programs are the Centers for Disease Control and Prevention, the Indian Health Service, The Health Resources and Services Administration and the Department of Veterans Affairs.

Many organizations outside of the government support diabetes research and education activities. These organizations include the American Diabetes Association (ADA), the Juvenile Diabetes Foundation International (JDFI), the American Association of Diabetes Educators (AADE), the Joslin Diabetes Center, the Barbara Davis Center for Childhood Diabetes, drug companies that develop diabetes products, and many other groups.

Advances in treatment and insulin delivery

In the past 15 years, advances in diabetes research have led to better ways to manage diabetes and treat its complications.

Major advances include

- New forms of purified insulin such as human insulin produced through genetic engineering.

- Rapid-acting insulin such as Humalog.

- Development of better ways for doctors to monitor blood glucose levels and for people with diabetes to test their own blood glucose levels at home.

- Development of external and implantable insulin pumps that deliver appropriate amounts of insulin, and which could replace daily injections.

- The use of laser treatment for diabetic eye disease, reducing the risk of blindness.

- Successful transplantation of kidneys in people whose own kidneys failed because of complications related to diabetes.

- Better ways of managing diabetic pregnancies, improving chances of a successful outcome.

- Development of new drugs to treat Type 2 diabetes and better ways to manage this form of the disease through weight control.

- Proof that intensive management of blood glucose levels reduces and may prevent development of microvascular complications of diabetes.

- Firm evidence that anti-hypertensive drugs called ACE-inhibitors prevent or delay kidney failure in people with diabetes.

- The development of the insulin pump as an alternative to daily insulin injections. The device, which is about the size of a beeper, draws on a pump reservoir, which is like a regular syringe filled with insulin. It operates on a small battery. A computer chip allows the user to control exactly how much insulin the pump delivers.

  The pump reservoir delivers insulin to the body via a thin plastic tube called an "infusion set." The infusion set has a needle or soft cannula at the end through which the insulin passes. The needle or cannula is inserted under the skin, usually on the abdomen. The infusion set is changed about every two or three days. The pump is intended to be used continuously and delivers insulin 24 hours a day according to a programmed plan unique to each pump wearer. This insulin keeps the blood glucose in the desired range between meals and through the night.

  The pump is not automatic. When food is eaten, the user programs the pump to deliver a "basal rate" of insulin matched to the amount of food that will be consumed. The pump user still needs to count carbohydrates and decide on the amount of insulin to be taken. Daily blood glucose monitoring is still required.

- The Personal Lasette, which uses a laser instead of a traditional lancet to obtain capillary blood samples for glucose monitoring. When the laser pulse is directed at a small area of the finger, it creates a tiny hole from which the blood is extracted via a precise, accurate beam of light that penetrates the skin without tearing it. The FDA has approved the Personal Lasette for home use by those over the age of five. A doctor's prescription is required in order to purchase this device. More information is available by calling the manufacturer at 800/846-0590 or by accessing the Web site at *www.cellrobotics.com.*

- The GlucoWatch, an alternative to glucose monitoring. On the back of the GlucoWatch is a pad that draws extra-cellular fluid from under the skin via a mild, battery-powered current. The glucose levels can be read on the watch, and it has a memory that allows you to keep track of your levels. You also can print out the values. An alarm can be set to warn you about low or high sugar levels. During the night, this watch can be used to help monitor blood sugar levels while sleeping. The GlucoWatch has not been approved by the FDA yet.

Inhaled insulin

A major breakthrough in diabetes treatment is the research on inhaled insulin. My son Joseph is participating in a nationwide study involving children ages 6 thru 11. He is in the group using the inhaler, which has eliminated the need for any extra injections due to high sugar levels.

The findings of an ongoing national study on inhaled insulin were revealed at the American Diabetes Association's 58th Annual Scientific Sessions in June 1998. Scientists and engineers from Inhale Therapeutic Systems designed the Inhale non-invasive deep-lung delivery system, which uses the combination of a proprietary dry powder formulation and processing.

The method for delivering insulin is similar to the way people with asthma take their medicine. The patient inhales a fine powder formulation of medicine from the inhaler pump, which is about the size of a 12-inch flashlight. The medicine reaches the deep lung tissue, then passes from the lungs into the bloodstream.

Before each inhalation, blood sugars must be evaluated. Patients will be able to use the pump anytime it is needed to lower blood sugar levels. Humalog is the only type of insulin that can be used with the inhaler at this time, so, in the morning and at bedtime, an NPH injection still will be needed.

The study looks very promising so far. The final trials will provide the evidence needed for the FDA to give its approval to mass-produce the medicine. I hope for everyone's sake that the inhaled insulin will be a reality on the market soon.

In the future

Research is ongoing to find the cause of diabetes as well as ways to prevent and cure the disease. Scientists are searching for genes that may be involved in both Type 1 and Type 2 diabetes. Some genetic and antibody markers for Type 1 have been identified, and it is now possible to screen relatives of people with Type 1 to determine whether they are at risk for diabetes.

Studies are underway to find drugs that stop the immune system from attacking the beta cells in order to prevent Type 1 diabetes from developing. Insulin is being given either orally or by injection to at-risk subjects in a nationwide, federally-funded DPT-1 trial in hopes of preventing the disease.

Transplantation of the pancreas or insulin-producing beta cells offers the best hope of a cure for people with Type 1 diabetes. Some successful pancreas transplants have been performed. However, people who have transplants must take powerful drugs that prevent rejection of the transplanted organ. These drugs are costly and may eventually cause serious health problems. Scientists are working to develop less harmful drugs and better methods of transplanting pancreatic tissue to prevent rejection or the reoccurrence of diabetes by the body.

Some methods under study include encapsulating the beta cells in a semipermeable membrane to protect them from immune attack; implanting the cells in the thymus gland as a way of inducing tolerance by the immune system; and using techniques of bio-engineering to create artificial beta cells that secrete insulin in response to glucose.

For Type 2 diabetes, the focus is on prevention. Approaches include identifying people at high risk for the disorder and encouraging them to lose weight, exercise more and maintain a healthy diet.

Resources

American Association of Diabetes Educators
100 W. Monroe
Suite 400
Chicago, IL 60603
800/832-6874
312/424-2426
www.aadenet.org

Provides information on diabetes education programs and a list of local Certified Diabetes Educators.

American Association of Oriental Medicine
433 Front Street
Catasauqua, PA 18032
888/500-7999
610/266-1433
www.aaom.org

Provides a list of local acupuncturists. All members of the organization have demonstrated competency in acupuncture and/or Oriental medicine.

American Diabetes Association
1701 N. Beauregard Street
Alexandria, VA 22311
800/232-3472
703/549-1500
www.diabetes.org

Provides information, support groups, funding for research, newsletters and "Diabetes Forecast" magazine. Local affiliates exist throughout the U.S. Also presents an African-American program at *www.diabetes.org/africanamerican*. This page also offers "The New Soul Food Cookbook for People with Diabetes." Information about diabetes camps is available by calling the ADA or logging onto *www.diabetes.org/ada/camps.htm*.

American Dietetic Association
216 West Jackson Boulevard
Suite 800
Chicago, IL 60606
800/877-1600
312/899-0040
www.eatright.org

Provides a list of local registered dietitians.

American Podiatric Medical Association (APMA)
9312 Old Georgetown Road
Bethesda, MD 20814-1698
800/366-8227
301/571-9200
www.apma.org

Provides materials regarding diabetes and the feet, including the booklet "Your Podiatric Physician Talks About Diabetes," along with many other brochures on various foot health topics.

Canadian Diabetes Association
15 Toronto Street, Suite 800
Toronto, ON M5C 2E3
Canada
800/BANTING (in Canada only)
416/363-3373
www.diabetes.ca
En français: *www.diabete.qc.ca*

The largest non-governmental supporter of diabetes research, education and advocacy in Canada.

Centers for Disease Control and Prevention (CDC)
Division of Diabetes Translation
National Center for Chronic Disease Prevention
   and Health Promotion
Mail Stop K-10
4770 Buford Highway, N.E.
Atlanta, GA 30341-3717
877/CDC-DIAB
770/488-5037
www.cdc.gov/health/diabetes.htm
En español: *www.cdc.gov/spanish/enfermedades/diabetes.htm*

Fact sheets, statistics, publications and information about state diabetes control programs. Several publications are available, including a patient guide in English or Spanish for people with diabetes, a diabetes surveillance report and an 8-page National Diabetes Fact Sheet.

ChildrenWithDiabetes.com
Diabetes123.com
www.childrenwithdiabetes.com/index_cwd.htm
www.Diabetes123.com

Both URLs lead to the same Web page for this on-line community, which was founded by the parent of a diabetic child. The site promotes understanding of the care and treatment of diabetes, especially in children; increases awareness of the need for unrestricted diabetes care for children at school and daycare; and supports families living with diabetes. Features information about school, research, chats, events and more, plus an on-line store. Free books and other items are listed when available. Provides a Q&A forum with over 30 healthcare professionals who answer diabetes questions that are sent to them via e-mail.

Diabetes Action Research and Education Foundation
426 C Street, N.E.
Washington, DC 20002
202/333-4520
www.daref.org

Supports and promotes education and scientific research to enhance the quality of life for all people affected by diabetes. Provides exercise videos designed for people with diabetes and publishes the booklet "Diabetes Self-Management: Basics and Beyond."

Diabetes Mall
1030 West Upas Street
San Diego, CA 92103
800/988-4772
619/497-0900
www.diabetesnet.com

An Internet-based source of information and retail products for diabetics. Offers a comprehensive weekly on-line diabetes newspaper called "Diabetes This Week," plus research reports, articles analyzing current diabetes issues, interactive tools for better blood sugar control, contests, information on the latest drugs, medications, devices, products, diets, blood sugar management tools and future developments in diabetes care. Also features an on-line store.

Diabetes Research Institute Foundation
3440 Hollywood Boulevard
Suite 100
Hollywood, FL 33021
954/964-4040
800/321-3437
www.drinet.org

An international center founded by parents of children with diabetes dedicated to the cure and treatment of the disease. The goal of the DRInet Web site is to make scientific research understandable by non-scientists. Has an informational and fun Web page just for kids at *www.drinet.org/html/kidzone.htm.*

Indian Health Service (IHS)
National Diabetes Program
5300 Homestead Road, N.E.
Albuquerque, NM 87110
505/248-4182
www.ihs.gov/medicalprograms/diabetes/

Develops, documents and sustains a health effort to prevent and control diabetes in American Indian and Alaska Native communities. Makes many diabetes resources available, including the Diabetes Curriculum Packet, nutrition education materials, general diabetes information, professional resources, training programs, posters, audiovisual materials and other patient education materials directed toward populations served by IHS. Materials can be obtained upon request from the IHS Diabetes Headquarters Office.

Institute for Health and Disability
University of Minnesota
P.O. Box 721
420 Delaware St., S.E.
Minneapolis, MN 55455
612/626-3087
www.cyfc.umn.edu/NRL/index.html

Provides comperehensive sources of information related to youths. Topics include psychosocial issues, disability awareness, developmental processes, family, education, cultural issues, advocacy and legal issues as well as health issues and more. Lists a bibliography of materials that can be found in libraries or purchased from bookstores or listed suppliers.

International Diabetic Athletes Association (IDAA)
1647 West Bethany Home Road
Suite B
Phoenix, AZ 85015
800/898-4322
602/433-2113
www.diabetes-exercise.org

Not just for athletes! The IDAA's mission is to enhance the quality of life for all people with diabetes through exercise. Offers "The Challenge," a quarterly newsletter. Also provides pamphlets on diabetes and exercise.

Joslin Diabetes Center
1 Joslin Place
Boston, MA 02215
800/547-5561
617/732-2415
www.joslin.org

A diabetes treatment research institution affiliated with Harvard Medical School, the Center is devoted to educating patients and professionals. Provides current diabetes news alerts on how to interpret information in the news media, the latest news about breakthroughs regarding diabetes, self-management training information, plus the opportunity to talk with others with diabetes and with health care professionals.

Juvenile Diabetes Foundation International
120 Wall Street
19th Floor
New York, NY 10005-4001
800/223-1138
212/785-9500
www.jdfcure.org

Not-for-profit, non-governmental organization for diabetes research founded in 1970 by parents of children with diabetes. JDF's priority is to find a cure for diabetes and its complications through the support of research. Provides information about local U.S. chapters, which offer information about diabetes, support groups and local fundraising events. Members receive "Countdown" magazine.

Maxishare
P.O. Box 2041
Milwaukee, WI 53201
800/444-7747

414/266-3428
www.maxishare.com

Offers pediatric educational materials, including brochures, videos and manuals for patients, families and caregivers.

National Diabetes Information Clearinghouse (NDIC)
One Information Way
Bethesda, MD 20892-3560
301/654-3327
www.niddk.nih.gov/health/diabetes/diabetes.htm
En español: *www.niddk.nih.gov/health/diabetes/diabetes.htm#spanish*

A service of NIDDK, the NDIC serves as a diabetes information, educational and referral resource for health professionals and the public. Makes diabetes education materials available for free or at little cost in both English and Spanish. Publishes the quarterly newsletter "Diabetes Dateline." Literature searches on a myriad of subjects related to diabetes are available.

National Eye Institute (NEI)
National Eye Health Education Program
2020 Vision Place
Bethesda, MD 20892-3655
301/496-5248
800/869-2020 (for health professionals only)
www.nei.nih.gov
En español: *www.nei.nih.gov/NDM_2000/s_facts.htm*

NEI's National Eye Health Education Program (NEHEP) promotes public and professional awareness of the importance of early diagnosis and treatment of diabetes eye diseases. NEI produces patient and professional education materials related to diabetic eye disease and its treatment, including literature for patients, guides for health professionals and education kits for community health workers and pharmacists. These titles focus on diabetic eye disease: Educating People with Diabetes (kit); Information Kit for Pharmacists; and, in Spanish, "Ojo con su Visión" ("Watch Out for Your Vision").

National Institute of Diabetes and Digestive and Kidney Diseases (NIDDK)
Office of Communication and Public Liason
31 Center Drive
MSC 2560
Bethesda, MD 20892-2560
301/654-3327
www.niddk.nih.gov/health/diabetes/diabetes.htm
En español: *www.niddk.nih.gov/health/diabetes/diabetes.htm#spanish*

The U.S. government's lead agency for diabetes research, NIDDK operates three clearinghouses that provide information regarding diabetes in both English and Spanish and funds six Diabetes Research and Training Centers.

National Institutes of Health (NIH)
9000 Rockville Pike
Rockville, MD 20892
301/496-4143
www.nih.gov
En español: *http://salud.nih.gov*

The NIH exists to improve the health of the American people. On-line databases are available, as well as directories and research reports.

National Kidney Foundation
30 E. 33rd Street
New York, NY 10016

800/622-9010
212/889-2210
www.kidney.org

The mission of the National Kidney Foundation is to prevent kidney and urinary tract diseases, to improve the health and well-being of individuals and families affected by these diseases and to increase the availability of all organs for transplantation. The Foundation provides continuing education of health care professionals as well as public education.

National Oral Health Information Clearinghouse (NOHIC)
One NOHIC Way
Bethesda, MD 20892-3500
301/402-7364
www.nidr.nih.gov

Serves as a resource for the public, patients and health professionals who seek information on the oral health of special-care patients. NOHIC provides a variety of services to help patients and professionals obtain information, including patient education materials and literature searches. "OH Notes" is NOHIC's annual newsletter.

New York Online Access to Health (NOAH)
www.noah.cuny.edu/illness/diabetes/diabetes.html
En español: *www.noah.cuny.edu/sp/illness/diabetes/spdiabetes.html*

This bilingual health information site is not restricted to New Yorkers. Offers a lot of diabetes facts in both English and Spanish.

Office of Minority Health Resource Center (OMH-RC)
P.O. Box 37337
Washington, DC 20013-7337

800/444-6472
www.omhrc.gov/omhrc/index.htm

Offers information, publications, mailing lists, database searches, referrals, scientific reports, journals and more for African-American, Alaska Native, Asian, Hispanic, Native American and Pacific Islander populations. OMH-RC publishes the newsletter "Closing the Gap."

Pritchett & Hull Associates Inc.
3440 Oakcliff Road, N.E.
Suite 110
Atlanta, GA 30340-3079
800/241-4925
770/451-0602
www.p-h.com

Publishes simple, readable patient education materials developed by health professionals. A catalog is available on the Web site.

Rick Mendosa's Diabetes Directory
www.mendosa.com
Non-English Resources: *www.mendosa.com/nonengl.htm*

Provides links to articles about diabetes topics in the news, plus a directory of diabetes Web sites. The Non-English Web Sites page offers resources for information about diabetes in many different languages.

Weight-Control Information Network (WIN)
1 WIN Way
Bethesda, MD 20892-3665
877/946-4627

202/828-1025
www.niddk.nih.gov/health/nutrit/win.htm

A national information service of the National Institutes of Health,
WIN offers fact sheets, pamphlets, article reprints, consensus state-
ments, reports, literature searches and videos on weight control,
obesity, and weight-related nutritional disorders. WIN's semi-an-
nual newsletter, "WIN Notes," provides health professionals with
the latest research findings and progress about the WIN program.

World Research Foundation
41 Bell Rock Plaza
Sedona, AZ 86351
520/284-3300
www.wrf.org/Diabetes.htm

International, non-profit health and environmental network that
provides information about various therapies used for diabetes.

Glossary

ADA – American Diabetes Association. Also, the American Diatetic Association.

Beta Cells – These cells are found in the islet of Langerhans in the pancreas. Beta cells make insulin.

Blood Glucose – Sugar level in the blood.

Blood Glucose Meter – A small machine that tests your blood glucose levels. When you place a small drop of blood on a strip that is inserted into the meter, it will calculate your blood glucose level and display a reading. It takes between 15 seconds and two minutes, depending on which meter you use.

Calorie – A unit of measurement of heat or energy provided by food. Carbohydrates, fats, protein, alcohol and sugar alcohols provide calories. Vitamins and minerals do not provide calories.

Carbohydrates – A group of compounds made up of starches or sugars that are a major source of energy for the body. Carbohydrates are prevalent in breads, cereals, fruits, and vegetables.

CHO – abbreviation for carbohydrates.

DCCT – Diabetes Control and Complications Trial.

Diabetes Mellitus – A disorder characterized by high levels of glucose in the blood. Diabetes Mellitus is caused by the failure of the body's pancreas to produce enough insulin.

DKA – Diabetic ketoacidosis.

Fats – A group of organic compounds that are composed of fatty acids. Fats are classified as either saturated or unsaturated. Unsaturated fats are classified as monounsaturated or polyunsaturated.

Fiber – Indigestible carbohydrates that are found in fruits, vegetables, and whole grains.

Food Exchange – List of foods with similar nutrient values that can be substituted, or exchanged, within the meal plan.

Free Foods – Food that contain few carbohydrates or calories and thus can be eaten freely (as much as the person desires). Generally, free foods have fewer than twenty calories per serving.

Fructose – A type of simple sugar that is found in fruits and honey.

Glucagon – A hormone produced by the pancreas that raises the blood sugar by stimulating the breakdown of glycogen.

Glucagon Injection Kit – A syringe filled with diluting solution, plus one vial of glucagon.

Glycogen – Stored form of carbohydrates in the liver; used as a reserve source of fuel.

Glucose – A simple sugar used by the body for energy.

Gram – A unit of weight and mass in the metric system. One ounce is equivalent to about 28 grams.

HDL – High Density Lipoproteins. This is the "good" type of cholesterol that protects against coronary heart disease.

Hyperglycemia – A condition in which abnormally high blood sugar levels exist. Some symptoms include frequent urination, increased thirst and mood changes.

Hypoglycemia – A condition in which the blood sugar level drops to an abnormally low level. Some symptoms include shakiness, confusion, headache, stomachache and cold sweats. Also called an insulin reaction.

IDDM – Insulin–dependent diabetes mellitus, or Type 1 disease (Autoimmune).

Insulin – A hormone that is produced by the pancreas to regulate the amount of sugar (glucose) in the bloodstream.

Insulin Resistance – When the body does not respond normally to the amount of insulin in the bloodstream, it produces increased amounts but still is unable to do the job of lowering the blood sugar after eating.

Ketoacidosis – Sometimes fatal complication of insulin dependent diabetes resulting from too little insulin in the body. There is an increase of ketones in the blood and an alteration of the body's acid-base balance. Ketoacidosis is an emergency situation that can result in a coma and death if left untreated.

Ketones – Acids produced when the body breaks down fat for energy. When there is not enough insulin in the body and these ketones cannot be utilized, they accumulate in the blood and spill into the urine. The amount of ketones can be measured in the urine using color strips or tablets.

LDL – Low–Density Lipoproteins. Cholesterol manufactured by the liver is carried through the bloodstream by LDL. High levels of LDL in the bloodstream can result in clogged arteries and heart disease. LDL is sometimes called the "bad" type of cholesterol.

Lactose – A sugar found naturally in milk.

Lancet – Used with the lancing device to prick the finger in order to obtain a blood sample for glucose monitoring.

NIDDK – National Institute of Diabetes and Digestive and Kidney Diseases.

Personal Lasette – A device that uses a laser pulse instead of a lancet to obtain capillary blood samples for glucose monitoring.

Polyunsaturated Fats – Oils from vegetable products that are liquid at room temperature. See HDL.

Protein – One of the three major sources of energy in the diet. Sources of protein include milk, eggs, fish, meats and some vegetables.

Retinopathy – Leakage from the eye's small blood vessels into the retina, which can cause blurred vision and other problems.

Saturated Fats – Oils from animal products. These are solid at room temperature. See LDL.

Sucralose – An artifical sweetener sold under the brand name Splenda. Sucralose is made made from sugar, but it is not recognized as sugar or carbohydrate by the body and contains no calories, so it can be used safely by diabetics.

Sucrose – A simple sugar processed from sugar cane and sugar beets.

Sugar – One of two types of carbohydrates, simple sugars come from milk, vegetables and fruits. Other simple sugars include table sugar and sugar alcohols.

Sugar Alcohols – Sorbitol, mannitol and xylitol are chemical substances that taste sweet but are absorbed more slowly by the body than simple sugars.

Urine Tests – A urine test measures the glucose or level of ketones in the urine.

Index